Wesley Hendricks

W9-CBC-083

The Inflammation Syndrome

Your Nutrition Plan for Great Health, Weight Loss, and Pain-Free Living

Completely Revised and Updated

Jack Challem

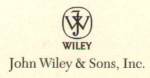

WILEY

John Wiley & Sons, Inc.

Copyright © 2010 by Jack Challem. All rights reserved

Published by John Wiley & Sons, Inc., Hoboken, New Jersey
Published simultaneously in Canada

The Inflammation Syndrome™ and Anti-Inflammation Syndrome™ are trademarks of Jack Challem.

Table on page 56 is from S. B. Eaton and S. B. Eaton II, "Paleolithic vs. Modern Diets—Selected Pathophysical Implications," *European Journal of Nutrition* 39, no. 2 (2000): 67–70. Reprinted with kind permission of Springer Springer & Business Media.

No part of this publication may be reproduced, stored in a retrieval system, or transmitted in any form or by any means, electronic, mechanical, photocopying, recording, scanning, or otherwise, except as permitted under Section 107 or 108 of the 1976 United States Copyright Act, without either the prior written permission of the Publisher, or authorization through payment of the appropriate per-copy fee to the Copyright Clearance Center, 222 Rosewood Drive, Danvers, MA 01923, (978) 750-8400, fax (978) 750-4470, or on the web at www.copyright.com. Requests to the Publisher for permission should be addressed to the Permissions Department, John Wiley & Sons, Inc., 111 River Street, Hoboken, NJ 07030, (201) 748-6011, fax (201) 748-6008, or online at http://www.wiley.com/go/permissions.

The information contained in this book is not intended to serve as a replacement for professional medical advice. Any use of the information in this book is at the reader's discretion. The author and the publisher specifically disclaim any and all liability arising directly or indirectly from the use or application of any information contained in this book. A health care professional should be consulted regarding your specific situation.

Designations used by companies to distinguish their products are often claimed as trademarks. In all instances where John Wiley & Sons, Inc., is aware of a claim, the product names appear in Initial Capital or ALL CAPITAL letters. Readers, however, should contact the appropriate companies for more complete information regarding trademarks and registration.

For general information about our other products and services, please contact our Customer Care Department within the United States at (800) 762-2974, outside the United States at (317) 572-3993 or fax (317) 572-4002.

Wiley also publishes its books in a variety of electronic formats. Some content that appears in print may not be available in electronic books. For additional information about Wiley products, visit our website at www.wiley.com.

Library of Congress Cataloging-in-Publication Data:

Challem, Jack.
   The inflammation syndrome : the complete nutritional program to prevent and reverse heart disease, arthritis, diabetes, allergies, and asthma / Jack Challem.—Rev. and expanded ed.
      p. cm.
   Includes bibliographical references and index.
   ISBN 978-0-470-44085-8 (pbk.)
   1. Inflammation—Diet therapy. 2. Inflammation—Alternative treatment. 3. Chronic diseases—Etiology. I. Title.
   RB131.C475 2010
   616'.0473—dc22

                                                                 2009037586

Printed in the United States of America
10 9 8 7 6 5

In memory of Harold G. Miller,
teacher, mentor, and friend

CONTENTS

FOREWORD

Occasional injuries are part of the human experience, and healing is the body's self-repair process. Healing begins with inflammation, which nature uses to clean up damaged tissues and protect against infection. So if inflammation is beneficial, why are so many modern diseases characterized by chronic and unhealthy inflammation?

This revised edition of *The Inflammation Syndrome* answers a major part of this important question. Chronic inflammation underscores and promotes virtually every disease, affecting millions of people, yet inflammation is also a symptom rather than the fundamental cause of these diseases. When we dig deeper, we find that chronic inflammation is the consequence of an injury to the body, combined with nutritional imbalances or deficiencies. To properly treat inflammatory diseases, it is essential to correct the underlying dietary problems.

We speak from experience. At the Center for the Improvement of Human Functioning International, physicians, nurses, and other staff members have focused on these objectives for more than thirty years. We use careful clinical and laboratory workups—what is now termed *evidence-based medicine*—to assess the health, nutritional reserves, and biochemical uniqueness of each patient. We have successfully treated people from around the country and around the world, many of whom were considered untreatable or incurable by conventional medicine.

Through these detailed individual workups, we have gained an understanding of chronic, or sustained, inflammation. More often than not, individuals with chronic inflammation, such as arthritis and asthma, have low levels of anti-inflammatory antioxidants (for example, vitamins E and C), omega-3 fatty acids, and other important nutrients. Many patients also have previously undetected adverse food reactions, abnormal gut permeability, yeast overgrowth, and hormonal imbalances. All of these factors can impair the normal functioning of the immune system, sustaining inflammation well beyond its biological usefulness.

The pharmaceutical perspective of inflammation focuses on relieving symptoms through over-the-counter analgesics and far more powerful prescription drugs. Inflammation does not result from a deficiency of aspirin, cortisone, or Cox-2 inhibitors. Rather, as *The Inflammation Syndrome* so well documents, there is a desperate need to address the basic nutritional influences on chronic inflammation. After all, no drug can ever make up for a nutritional deficiency. Under these circumstances, it becomes paramount to nourish a person's biochemistry with the best nutrition.

This is where measuring a patient's nutrient levels proves to be so helpful in confirming the underlying nutritional and biochemical causes of inflammation and in motivating patients to act. It would be easy to lecture a patient on the anti-inflammatory effects of good nutrition, omega-3 fatty acids (which include fish oils), or vitamin E. But a far more powerful motivator is testing and demonstrating the patient's low levels of specific nutrients.

By doing so, we have found time and again that such hard evidence is extremely persuasive. This meaningful individual information, combined with the ease of making dietary improvements and taking supplements, empowers patients with knowledge and motivates them to undertake self-healing. Patients develop the attitude "I want my levels to be optimal," and then they work toward achieving them. Furthermore, from our medical perspective, laboratory testing enables us to later recheck nutrient values to confirm proper absorption and utilization.

Through testing, we have realized that no one can ever assume that a person's diet is adequate. For example, a cardiac surgeon would never simply hope his patient's potassium level is sufficient to prevent fatal arrhythmias during heart surgery; he ensures that it is. The same approach applies to the treatment of chronic inflammation. To achieve optimal levels of many nutrients, one must often consume amounts of vitamins, minerals, and other nutrients greater than those "officially" recommended for health. There is nothing wrong in doing so, especially when tests have shown patients to be low in these nutrients. At the very least, erring on the side of modest excess provides a margin of safety, a dose of nutritional insurance.

Jack Challem, the author of *The Inflammation Syndrome*, is a gifted health writer with a profound understanding of the role good nutrition plays in health. He has written a sound and practical book of benefit to anyone with chronic inflammation. As we read and discussed his book, we visualized Jack working in a huge lighthouse. The light being emitted is the cumulative scientific evidence so deftly organized and clearly presented here. The danger is the jagged rocks of chronic, sustained inflammation, which underlie almost every serious health issue facing modern society—and the reason for the lighthouse. All of us—readers, patients, and physicians alike—are piloting our own boats and, as a society, we are heading for the rocks. Will we see the light? Can we avoid the forces making us drift in the dark? To survive, we must rediscover the great Hippocratic ideal: Let food be thy medicine.

—Ronald E. Hunninghake, M.D.
Medical Director
The Olive W. Garvey Center for Healing Arts
Wichita, Kansas

—Hugh D. Riordan, M.D.
Founder
The Center for the Improvement of
Human Functioning International, Inc.
Wichita, Kansas

ACKNOWLEDGMENTS

Many individuals made major and minor contributions to my thinking on inflammation and to this updated edition of *The Inflammation Syndrome*.

My good friend Ron Hunninghake, M.D., has often brainstormed with me on the role of diet in inflammation and many other health topics. In the course of our numerous discussions, we've helped shape each other's views of inflammatory diseases, and I am appreciative of his time and friendship. The work of many other people, such as Björn Falck Madsen, Søren Mavrogenis, Melissa Diane Smith, Ashton and Matt Embry, the late Abram Hoffer, M.D., Ph.D., and others, has also contributed to my views on eating habits and supplements.

I want to thank my previous literary agent, the late Michael Cohn, and my current agent, Jack Scovil, for their support in getting my ideas published. I also thank my editor, Tom Miller, who has always encouraged me to clarify and simplify the complexities of health and self-help. I would also like to thank Kimberly Monroe-Hill and Patricia Waldygo for their careful editing of this book.

Finally, I thank my nutrition coaching clients and my many fans and readers, whose positive feedback always brightens my days.

Introduction
to the Original Edition

One condition explains your stiff fingers, aching muscles, and arthritic joints. One condition lies at the root of your troublesome allergies and asthma. And one condition describes the underlying cause of heart disease, Alzheimer's disease, and some types of cancer.

It is *inflammation*.

As you read this, medicine is rapidly redefining coronary artery (heart) disease, the leading cause of death among people in the United States and most other Westernized nations, as an inflammatory disease of the blood vessels. Physicians are quickly adopting a new and inexpensive blood test—high-sensitivity C-reactive protein—to measure their patients' level of inflammation and risk of suffering a heart attack. And as the evidence mounts, physicians and medical researchers are recognizing that other major chronic diseases are fueled by inflammation as well.

Most of us understand inflammation as something that causes redness, tenderness, stiffness, and pain. It is the core of inflammatory "-itis" disease, and it also is intertwined in every disease, including obesity, diabetes, and multiple sclerosis.

Inflammation is why professional athletes and weekend warriors often development muscle aches. It is why some people's gums bleed whenever they brush their teeth. And it is why some people develop stomach ulcers.

1

Despite their different symptoms, all of these health problems are united by the same thread: they have runaway inflammation in common.

And as you may well realize, many people suffer from more than one inflammatory disorder. This constellation of related diseases, such as the combination of heart disease, arthritis, and periodontitis, can best be described as the Inflammation Syndrome.

—⚬—

Estimated Number of North Americans with Some Inflammatory Diseases

Millions of North Americans suffer from inflammatory disorders, some of which have only recently been recognized as inflammatory in nature:

Allergic and nonallergic rhinitis	39 million
Asthma	17 million
Cardiovascular diseases	60 million
Arthritis (all types combined)	70 million
Osteoarthritis	21 million
Rheumatoid arthritis	2 million

—⚬—

Everyone experiences inflammation at one time or another, and we actually need it to survive. But *chronic inflammation* is a sign that something has gone seriously awry with your health. Instead of protecting and healing, chronic inflammation breaks down your body and makes you older and more frail.

Most people treat inflammation with one or more over-the-counter or prescription drugs. At best these drugs temporarily mask the symptoms of inflammation, not treat its underlying causes. Worse, the side effects of these drugs can often be extraordinarily dangerous, causing weight gain, severe stomach pain, bone deformities, and heart failure.

Unfortunately, a physician's diagnosis of many -itis diseases, such as dermatitis or gastritis, is often meaningless. The doctor might feel proud of his diagnosis, but it is merely a description of the symptoms, not of its cause.

To understand the cause of the modern epidemic of inflammatory diseases, we have to look at how the average person's diet has deteriorated over the past two or three generations. The bottom line is that the foods you eat have a powerful bearing on your health and, specifically, inflammation.

How does food influence your inflammation, your aches and pains?

Your body is a remarkable biological machine, designed to make an assortment of pro- and anti-inflammatory substances. What you eat—proteins, carbohydrates, fats, vitamins and vitaminlike nutrients, and minerals—provides the nutritional building blocks of these substances. Some nutrients help form your body's inflammation-promoting compounds, which normally help fight infections. Others help produce your body's anti-inflammatory substances, which moderate and turn off inflammation.

Until recently, people ate a relative balance of pro- and anti-inflammatory nutrients. Today, because of extensive food processing, our diet has become seriously unbalanced. The typical Western diet now contains at least thirty times more of pro-inflammatory nutrients than just a century ago. As a result, people have become nutritionally and biochemically primed for powerful, out-of-control inflammatory reactions. An injury, infection, or sometimes nothing more than age-related wear and tear create the spark that, in a manner of speaking, sets your body on fire.

The Inflammation Syndrome reveals many of the hidden dangers in foods that set the stage for inflammation, worsen aches and pains, and increase the long-term risk of debilitating and life-threatening diseases. This book explains how and why inflammation eats away at your health.

For example:

- Common cooking oils, such as corn, safflower, and soy oils, can make arthritis and asthma worse.
- Fries and other deep-fried foods, breakfast bars, and cookies can interfere with your body's innate ability to control inflammation.
- Corn-fed beef, promoted as healthy, is far worse than grass-fed beef and can aggravate your inflammation.
- Not eating your vegetables or taking your vitamins can increase breathing problems in people with asthma.
- Being overweight increases your body's production of inflammation-causing substances.
- Taking common anti-inflammatory drugs will actually make your osteoarthritis far worse.
- If you have one inflammatory disease, you are likely to develop others in the coming years, because the inflammation will eventually spread and affect other parts of your body.

I have had my own experience with inflammation and how I have avoided chronic pain. Several years ago, while in the British Museum in London, I paid careful attention to a sign reading "Mind the Step." Unfortunately for me, the area was not well lit and the sign failed to warn me of a second step. I tripped and seriously injured my right foot. The pain was so excruciating that I almost passed out. I sat down while my head cleared and, I had hoped, for the pain to ease.

It didn't. By the next morning, my entire foot was literally turning black and blue. Although no bones were broken, I did give myself one of the most serious types of muscle strain. A couple of days later, on the next leg of my trip, in France, I hobbled around at a scientific conference on antioxidant vitamins. Climbing into the shower was an ordeal, as was putting on my socks and shoes. My foot had swelled, its color was awful, and I was taking aspirin several times daily to reduce the inflammation, swelling, and pain.

Weeks later, at home, my foot had regained its normal color and, by all outward signs, had healed. However, I still felt a sharp pain in the foot whenever I walked. I realized that this injury, if it did not heal soon and properly, could lead to a lifetime of chronic inflammation and pain. Frustratingly, all of the vitamin supplements I had been taking for years didn't seem to help. And then it dawned on me. That scientific meeting in France was about a well-known herbal antioxidant made from French maritime pine bark (called Pycnogenol), and the scientific literature showed it to have powerful anti-inflammatory effects. I started taking it, and within days the pain went away. To rule out the power of suggestion, I stopped taking the supplement for a few days, and the pain returned. I started taking the supplement again and the inflammation and pain went away and have never returned. I walk and hike long distances without any discomfort in the foot.

The Inflammation Syndrome does not simply dwell on the problem of inflammation. Most of this book coaches you on how to avoid the foods that make you more susceptible to inflammation and to instead select foods that can reduce inflammation and your risk of many diseases. *The Inflammation Syndrome* describes a new way of viewing inflammatory disorders as a consequence of eating an unbalanced diet.

You will learn plenty of practical information about how to prevent and reverse inflammation. The book's Anti-Inflammation [AI] Syndrome Diet Plan describes

- the dietary imbalances that lead to chronic inflammation;
- a balanced, nutritious diet plan to reduce inflammation;

- tasty recipes and guidelines for making your own anti-inflammatory meals;
- the best natural anti-inflammation supplements, such as fish oils, vitamin E, herbs, and many others;
- case histories of patients treated by nutritionally oriented practitioners.

You may wonder why you should trust the advice of someone who is not a physician.

The reason is simple, though it may surprise you: while I believe the majority of physicians are sincere and well-meaning, most do not understand the fundamental role of nutrition in health. Medical schools teach virtually nothing about the practical, preventive, and therapeutic uses of nutrition and supplements. The doctors I write about in this book are notable exceptions to this rule in that they are both sincere *and* have an understanding of nutrition.

For more than twenty-five years, I have been reading scientific and medical journals; talking with nutritionally oriented biologists, biochemists, and physicians; and writing about how vitamins, minerals, and other aspects of nutrition can greatly improve health. I have also published original research articles in medical journals, something rare for nutrition writers. Though I am not a medical scientist, I have a solid understanding of the science behind the health benefits of nutrition and supplements.

In many ways, *The Inflammation Syndrome* expands on the concepts described in my previous book *Syndrome X: The Complete Nutritional Program to Prevent and Reverse Insulin Resistance.* Far more than genes, poor eating habits are at the core of most modern degenerative disorders, including chronic inflammation. *The Inflammation Syndrome* is supported by hundreds of scientific studies and by successful clinical experiences, many of which you will read. Some of my scientific references are at the back of this book, and I encourage you to share all of them with your physician. [As of the revised edition, the references have been moved to www.inflammationsyndrome.com.]

Ultimately, you alone are responsible for your own health. You cannot ignore your personal responsibility and simply turn your body over to a doctor the way you might ask a mechanic to fix your car. This book provides a plan for you to empower yourself to safely prevent and overcome inflammatory disorders. You will discover how easy it is to take charge of your diet and your health—and to feel better than you ever imagined.

Introduction
to the Revised Edition

When *The Inflammation Syndrome* was first published early in 2003, it proposed what was then a bold and audacious idea—that many different types of inflammatory diseases were related to one another. Today, this idea is widely accepted.

Indeed, a great deal has changed over the last few years, necessitating this updated edition of the book. First, inflammation is now recognized as an undercurrent in all disease processes. Second, inflammation (not cholesterol) is now understood to be the primary determining factor in coronary heart disease, which is the leading cause of death in most developed countries, although many doctors are yet to act on this knowledge. Third, inflammatory disorders—for example, allergies, arthritis, heart disease, and inflammatory bowel disease, to name but a few—share common causes and also increase the risk of developing other inflammatory diseases.

What events have led to such dramatic changes in the perception of inflammation?

Medical thinking about the role of inflammation in disease began to broaden in the late 1990s, following the development and increased use of the high-sensitivity C-reactive protein (hsCRP) test. The test was revolutionary in that it could measure subtle, low-grade inflammation—the type of inflammation that is not always obvious but that slowly breaks down the body and leads to chronic degenerative diseases. Researchers at Harvard Medical School showed that chronic low-grade inflammation was a major factor in the development of heart disease and, just as important, that the CRP test could identify people who were at risk of suffering a heart attack. In fact, high levels of CRP are a far better predictor of heart attack risk than is cholesterol.

It didn't take long before other researchers began to look for elevated CRP levels in other diseases. What they found was fascinating and further shifted medical thinking about the role of inflammation in disease. For example, people who are overweight or have type 2 diabetes typically have elevated CRP levels. Being overweight and having type 2 diabetes are major risk factors for heart disease, another proof of the disease linkage that forms the inflammation syndrome. Almost everyone with type 2 diabetes is overweight, and fat cells (particularly those that form around the waistline) secrete inflammation-producing compounds, including interleukin-6 (IL-6) and CRP.

—⚊—

The Prevalence of Some Inflammatory Diseases in North America

How has the prevalence of inflammatory diseases changed since the first edition of *The Inflammation Syndrome* was published in 2003? Compare the numbers below with those on page 2.

Allergic and nonallergic rhinitis	39 million
Asthma	22 million
Cardiovascular diseases	60 million
Arthritis (all types)	70 million
Osteoarthritis	21 million
Rheumatoid arthritis	2 million
Diabetes/prediabetes	100 million
Overweight/obesity	120 million
Cancers	3.4 million (30% of all cancers)
Rhinitis	56 million
Gingivitis	270 million
Sinusitis	40 million
Inflammation syndrome	250 million (estimated)

—⚊—

At the same time, there has been a surge in research on natural anti-inflammatory substances, such as certain foods, herbs and spices, and supplements, and my discussion of these substances forms the core of *The Inflammation Syndrome*. Here's the good news: you can use these natural substances to safely reduce inflammation and pain and restore your health.

What's new in this edition of *The Inflammation Syndrome*?

- I have updated much of the information throughout the book, based on recent scientific and medical research. (To save space, my references appear at www.inflammationsyndrome.com.)
- I have simplified many of my recommendations to make them more practical and easier to follow. For example, companies market dozens of anti-inflammatory supplements, but I have focused on the ones most strongly supported by scientific research. I also recommend specific brands of products (which I tended to avoid doing in the past), to make purchasing decisions easier for you.
- I discuss several natural anti-inflammatory substances produced by the body that have been discovered since I wrote the first edition of this book. These remarkable compounds include *resolvins*, *protectins*, and *lipoxins*, and the body makes them from healthy dietary fats. Their activity can be increased through both diet and supplements.
- I explain the research that demonstrates the benefits of curcumin, one of the most powerful natural anti-inflammatory compounds. Curcumin is an extract of the spice turmeric, and the latest research indicates that it blocks ninety-seven different inflammatory mechanisms in the body—more than any other natural or synthetic substance.
- I also discuss at length the anti-inflammatory properties of another natural compound, Pycnogenol. Long known for its cardiovascular effects, this extract of French maritime pine bark has impressive and scientifically documented anti-inflammatory benefits.
- In the first edition of *The Inflammation Syndrome*, I explained how gamma-linolenic acid (a plant oil) has a potent anti-inflammatory action and is synergistic with the inflammation-quenching omega-3 fish oils. Over the last few years, researchers have documented still more health benefits from gamma-linolenic acid, and I have included a discussion of these.

- Similarly, the research on the health benefits of omega-3 fish oils has amounted to a medical landslide. Almost every week, medical and scientific journals report new advantages of consuming fish oils. I have included more recent and comprehensive information on omega-3 fish oils.
- I also include information on vitamin D, which has emerged as an immune-modulating and anti-inflammatory nutrient, and on many other nutrients you may lack in your diet.
- There's much more in the updated edition of *The Inflammation Syndrome*, such as new recipes for tasty anti-inflammatory meals.

Before you read further, I would like to share three brief case histories about how *The Inflammation Syndrome* has helped people regain their health and their lives.

Susan had long suffered with frightening episodes of asthma. Like many other people, she had gone from doctor to doctor, and then a specialist (a pulmonologist) prescribed several different medications to control her asthmatic symptoms. She still had to use a steroid-containing inhaler several times a day. After she followed the advice in *The Inflammation Syndrome* for only one month, her symptoms decreased, and now she often goes an entire week without having to use the inhaler. Susan has also been able to reduce her other medications.

Deirdre had dealt with the crippling symptoms of Epstein-Barr infection and inflammatory pain for years. After reading *The Inflammation Syndrome*, she added gamma-linolenic acid supplements to her regimen—without making any changes to her diet—and nearly all of her muscle and joint pain disappeared. Her initial success motivated Deirdre to take other supplements, including vitamins C and E, and then to make important dietary changes. She has had such a dramatic recovery that she now recommends a similar program to her relatives.

When Jennifer read *The Inflammation Syndrome*, everything about her health and that of her family suddenly made sense. She weighed more than three hundred pounds and had type 2 diabetes. She and other family members had allergies, a brother and a sister had inflammatory bowel disease, and her mother had ulcers. Jennifer felt better within several days of beginning to follow my dietary recommendations and e-mailed me: "This book has changed my life!" Jennifer has a lot of health issues to deal with, but she's on the right track and was quickly able to start walking without her cane.

These are some of the many success stories I've heard from readers. These people have been successful in large part because, for the first time in their lives, they've been able to "connect the dots" in their inflammatory disorders—and then take small and big steps toward regaining their health. You can, too!

PART I

The Inflammation-
Disease Connection

CHAPTER 1

Meet the Inflammation Syndrome

The Inflammation Syndrome Helps Janet Make
Sense of Her Health Problems

Janet was in her midforties and felt worn down and much older because of a growing list of health problems. She was overweight and prediabetic and had high blood pressure, allergies, inflammatory bowel disease, rosacea, gastric reflux, and morning aches and pains. Janet was taking seven different prescription drugs that had marginal, if any, benefits—but that did zap her energy levels.

Her life wasn't getting better, it was getting worse. And as she looked at her parents and older sisters, she could see her future: a debilitating combination of diseases that forced her parents into early retirement and that led to long-term disability for her sisters. Tough-minded and tenacious, Janet didn't want to follow in her family's footsteps.

As she searched for a solution, she found a nutritionally oriented physician who understood that eating habits had a strong bearing on health and disease risk. He ordered Janet to undergo blood tests for nutrient levels, food allergies, and high-sensitivity C-reactive protein (hsCRP), an indicator of chronic low-grade inflammation.

His diagnosis stunned Janet. Her vitamin C and D levels were low, she was sensitive to wheat and dairy products, and she had high blood levels of hsCRP. Chronic inflammation was underlying most of Janet's health problems. "I was a disaster—and an even bigger disaster waiting to happen," she said.

The doctor explained how Janet's health problems were related to one another, and he outlined a new approach to eating that focused on high-quality proteins (such as fish and chicken) and high-fiber, non-starchy vegetables (for example, salad greens and steamed broccoli and cauliflower). He suggested that Janet avoid all packaged foods containing wheat and dairy products. On the doctor's advice, Janet began to take a number of supplements, including vitamins C and D, anti-inflammatory omega-3 fish oils, and an anti-inflammatory plant oil called gamma-linolenic acid.

By the end of the first week, Janet's energy levels were higher than they had been in years, and her general sense of well-being had increased considerably. By the end of Janet's second week on the anti-inflammatory diet and supplements, she had lost seven pounds and her gastric reflux had stopped. Even though it was springtime and the height of allergy season for Janet, her nasal symptoms were relatively mild. After one month, most of Janet's symptoms had either diminished or disappeared, and, working with her doctor, she was able to cease taking most of her medications. She also continued to lose weight.

"I'm a new person," she said. "I had forgotten what it was like to feel good and energized about life."

Even if you seem to be pretty healthy today, there's a good chance that inflammation is simmering in your body, quietly damaging your heart, your mind, and other tissues. Such inflammation may be stirred up by physical injuries, by frequent colds and flus, allergies, by eating the wrong types of fats and carbohydrates, and by having a "spare tire" around your middle. At a certain point, your inflammation will boil over into painful and debilitating symptoms.

Inflammation is a normal process that can go dreadfully wrong. It is supposed to protect us from infections and promote healing when we are injured.

Yet chronic inflammation does just the opposite: it breaks down our bodies and makes us more susceptible to disease. Inflammation forces millions of people with arthritis to alter their daily lives, and it compels millions of people with asthma to be cautious because they do not know when their next suffocating attack will occur. Millions of other people—

with multiple sclerosis, lupus, diabetes, and other disorders—also suffer from chronic inflammation.

The Inflammation Syndrome

Individual inflammatory disorders such as asthma or rheumatoid arthritis are bad enough. Far more insidious is the inflammation syndrome, the significance of which is only now being recognized in medical circles.

A syndrome is a group of symptoms that characterizes a particular disorder. For example, in my earlier book *Syndrome X: The Complete Nutritional Program to Prevent and Reverse Insulin Resistance*, Syndrome X was defined as a combination of abdominal fat, insulin resistance, hypertension, and elevated cholesterol—all of which significantly increase the risk of diabetes and coronary artery disease.

Similarly, the inflammation syndrome reflects the coexistence of at least two (and often more) inflammatory disorders that greatly increase the risk of developing more serious inflammatory diseases. What causes this ongoing buildup of inflammation? Although an inflammatory response may primarily affect specific tissues, such as the knees, it frequently radiates through the body and attacks other tissues. Over a number of years this systemic (bodywide) inflammation contributes to diseases that might appear unrelated but that do share a common thread of chronic inflammation.

Some examples of the inflammation syndrome are in order. Let's start with being overweight, a condition that affects two-thirds of Americans and growing numbers of people in most other developed countries.

Excess weight contributes to inflammation because fat cells secrete chemicals, such as interleukin-6 and C-reactive protein, that promote inflammation. Being overweight increases the risk of developing many other diseases, and part of the reason is related to the undercurrent of inflammation. If you are overweight, you have a greater risk of developing adult-onset (that is, type 2) diabetes, which also has a strong inflammatory component. Inflammation in diabetes is related to being overweight, to having elevated blood sugar and insulin levels, and to consuming too many refined carbohydrates (such as white bread and sugary breakfast cereals).

The inflammation syndrome does not stop here. Having diabetes also heightens your chances of suffering from periodontitis, a type of dental inflammation. Each of these disorders—overweight, diabetes, and periodontitis—is serious by itself. But as the inflammation in these disorders simmers year after year, it also increases the risk of developing coronary artery disease, which medicine has recently recognized as an inflammatory disease of the blood vessels. In a nutshell, each inflammatory disorder has an additive effect, aggravating the body's overall level of inflammation and the risk of succumbing to very serious diseases.

Other examples of the inflammation syndrome abound. Allergies stir up the inflammatory response, which may give rise to rheumatoid arthritis, an autoimmune (self-allergic) disease. Infections also trigger an immune response, and chronic infections and inflammation account for an estimated 30 percent of cancers. Joint injuries frequently put an inflammatory response into motion, setting the stage for osteoarthritis. Serious head injuries and their resultant brain inflammation increase the long-term risk of developing Alzheimer's disease, which is also being viewed by doctors as an inflammatory process affecting brain cells.

This is serious and scary stuff, and the stakes for your health are very high. But the point of this book is to teach you that chronic inflammation and the inflammation syndrome can be prevented and reversed.

—⁂—

Connecting the Dots in the Inflammation Syndrome

Unless inflammatory problems are controlled or reversed, they tend to get worse, creating a cascade that leads to more serious inflammatory diseases, such as coronary heart disease and Alzheimer's. This list describes the greater risks associated with certain inflammatory disorders.

- Obesity boosts the risk of developing diabetes.
- Obesity and diabetes set the stage for coronary heart disease.
- Diabetes increases the likelihood of macular degeneration and cataracts.
- Joint injuries often lead to osteoarthritis.
- Brain injuries increase the chances of developing Alzheimer's disease.
- Periodontal disease heightens the risk of getting coronary heart disease.
- Allergies can aggravate the pulmonary system and may give rise to asthma.
- Allergies increase the odds of suffering from autoimmune disorders.

- Rheumatoid arthritis may bring about conditions that promote coronary heart disease.
- Chronic inflammation increases the risk of getting cancer.
- Gastritis may eventually result in gastric cancer.
- Inflammatory bowel disease increases the risk of developing osteoporosis.

—w—

What Is Chronic Inflammation?

Inflammation assumes many different forms, and everyone experiences it at one time or another. The most familiar type of inflammation is sudden and acute, such as when you burn yourself in the kitchen, overuse your muscles while moving furniture, or injure your tendons when playing sports. The injured area swells, turns red, and becomes tender to the touch.

Under normal circumstances inflammation helps you heal, and it can even save your life. For example, if you accidentally cut your finger with a knife, bacteria from the knife, the air, or the surface of your skin immediately penetrate the breach. Unchecked, these bacteria would quickly spread through your bloodstream and kill you.

Your body's immune system almost immediately recognizes these bacteria as foreign, however, and unleashes a coordinated attack to contain and stop the infection. Inflammation encourages tiny blood vessels in your finger to dilate, allowing a variety of white blood cells to leak out, track, and engulf bacteria. Some of these white blood cells also pick up and destroy cells damaged by the cut. In addition, inflammation signals the body to grow new cells to seal the cut. Within a day or two, your cut finger becomes less inflamed, and a few days later, it is completely healed.

Your body responds in similar fashion if you strain a muscle, for example, when you lift too heavy a box or overexert yourself during sports. The resulting inflammation, characterized by swelling, pain, and stiffness, is designed to remove damaged muscle cells and help initiate the healing process to replace those cells. Again, within a few days the inflammation decreases and you are well on the road to recovery.

Chronic inflammation, however, is very different. It does not go away, at least not quickly, and many people believe from their own experience that it will never go away. It results in persistent swelling, stiffness, or pain. Furthermore, you have a greater susceptibility to inflammation as you age, but that, too, may be reversible.

—∞—

The Inflammation Syndrome Quiz

Many people know that they regularly experience inflammation—the pain, stiffness, and swelling are obvious signs. Yet other people interpret stiffness and pain as vague signs of not being in good health, or they don't connect their use of certain drugs (such as ibuprofen and aspirin) to inflammatory diseases or the inflammation syndrome. This quiz is designed to help you make those connections. Circle Y (yes) or N (no) for each item or question.

Do you have any of the following health problems or issues?

AIDS or HIV infection	Y/N
Allergies (any type)	Y/N
Arthritis (any type)	Y/N
Asthma	Y/N
Blood sugar (elevated)	Y/N
Bronchitis	Y/N
Cancer	Y/N
Celiac disease or gluten intolerance	Y/N
Coronary artery (heart) disease	Y/N
Chronic obstructive pulmonary disease	Y/N
Chronic fatigue syndrome	Y/N
Dark circles or puffiness under the eyes	Y/N
Diabetes	Y/N
Diverticulitis	Y/N
Cholesterol (elevated)	Y/N
Fibromyalgia	Y/N
Food cravings (e.g., chocolate, carbs)	Y/N
Forgetfulness	Y/N

Gingivitis or periodontitis	Y/N
Glucose intolerance	Y/N
Heartburn or gastric reflux	Y/N
Hepatitis	Y/N
Inflammatory bowel disease	Y/N
Irritability	Y/N
Eczema or psoriasis	Y/N
Lupus	Y/N
Metabolic syndrome (or Syndrome X)	Y/N
Multiple sclerosis	Y/N
Obesity	Y/N
Prediabetes	Y/N
Sinusitis	Y/N
Sleep apnea	Y/N
Stomach ulcers	Y/N
Ulcerated varicose veins	Y/N

Interpretation: These health issues have either strong or subtle links to inflammation. If you have answered yes to more than one of these health issues, you may have signs of inflammation syndrome.

Do you have any of the following symptoms?

Do you bruise easily?	Y/N
Does your body feel stiff when you get out of bed in the morning?	Y/N
Do you have any stiff or aching joints, such as those in your fingers or knees?	Y/N
Do you have frequent backaches?	Y/N
Do you have frequent muscle aches?	Y/N
Do you experience premenstrual syndrome (PMS)?	Y/N
Are you overweight, and is some or all of this excess weight around your belly?	Y/N
Is your nose stuffy or runny a lot of the time or during certain seasons?	Y/N
Do you suffer injuries from falls or from bumping into objects?	Y/N

Have you been hospitalized for surgery during the
 last twelve months?   Y/N

Do you get frequent colds or flus?   Y/N

Do you have any skin sores, cuts, or rashes that don't
 seem to heal?   Y/N

Do you tend to feel tired after you eat, particularly after
 lunch and dinner?   Y/N

When you were younger, did you experience a lot of
 athletic injuries?   Y/N

Interpretation: Answering yes to any of these questions suggests that you are dealing with inflammation, although it may not always be obvious.

Do you take any of the following medications once or more each week?

Aspirin   Y/N

Ibuprofen (e.g., Advil, Motrin)   Y/N

Acetaminophen (e.g., Tylenol)   Y/N

Naproxen sodium (e.g., Aleve)   Y/N

Any other kind of over-the-counter drug to reduce pain Y/N

Celebrex or any other kind of prescription drug to reduce pain Y/N

Lipitor, Zocor, or another cholesterol-lowering drug Y/N

Corticosteroid drugs (e.g., cortisone or prednisone) Y/N

Interpretation: Most of these drugs are used to reduce inflammation and pain. Frequent use indicates that you are trying to ease the inflammation symptoms but are not addressing the underlying causes.

Do you take any of the following dietary supplements (other than the amounts found in a multivitamin), or have you found that they reduce any of the symptoms you have indicated?

Omega-3 fish oils   Y/N

Gamma-linolenic acid   Y/N

Glucosamine or chondroitin   Y/N

Herbal products, including curcumin, devil's claw, green tea,
 mushrooms, Pycnogenol, grape-seed extract, quercetin,
 Saint-John's-wort, ginseng, ginkgo biloba, or any others Y/N

Interpretation: Many people take these supplements to reduce inflammation and pain. If you do, you may already be on the right track.

These questions are about your cooking and eating habits at home.

Do you, or does your spouse or domestic partner, cook mostly
with corn, peanut, sunflower, safflower, or soybean oil
(as opposed to olive oil)? Y/N

Do you eat prepackaged microwave meals for breakfast,
lunch, or dinner more than once a week? Y/N

Of the foods you've eaten at home during the last week,
would you estimate that half or more came from boxes,
cans, bottles, or jars (as opposed to being fresh vegetables,
chicken, fish, or meat)? Y/N

When you eat at home, do you use bottled salad dressings? Y/N

Do you eat pasta, bread, white rice, or pizza (one, some, or
all three) daily? Y/N

Do you eat potatoes (baked, mashed, French fries) once
or more a week? Y/N

Do you eat cookies, ice cream, cakes, doughnuts, brownies,
candy, or pastries at least once a week? Y/N

Do you use margarine instead of butter? Y/N

Do you eat a lot of ground beef (e.g., burgers)? Y/N

Do you dislike eating most vegetables? Y/N

Do you dislike eating fish? Y/N

Do you consume regular (sweetened) soft drinks or add
sugar to your coffee or tea? Y/N

Do you really enjoy eating tomatoes, potatoes, eggplant,
or chile peppers? Y/N

Do you eat pork more than once a week? Y/N

Interpretation: If you have answered yes to one or more of these questions, your dietary habits likely promote inflammation.

These questions are about your eating habits at restaurants.

Do you eat at fast-food restaurants (e.g., McDonald's, Burger
King, KFC, Taco Bell, or others) once or more each week? Y/N

Do you consume soft drinks?	Y/N
Do you eat pasta or pizza in a restaurant at least once a week?	Y/N
Do you eat breaded and fried chicken, shrimp, or fish more than once a month?	Y/N
Do you like barbecue sauces on your food?	Y/N
Do you eat French fries?	Y/N
Do you eat at a Chinese restaurant more than once a week?	Y/N

Interpretation: If you have answered yes to one or more of these questions, your dietary habits likely promote inflammation.

—◊—

Recognizing Inflammatory Disorders

Physicians often speak in their own language, but it is actually very easy to identify most inflammatory diseases when you hear them referred to in conversation or read about them. Inflammatory diseases usually end with the suffix "-itis." For example, gastritis means inflammation of the stomach, tendinitis refers to inflammation of the tendons, and gingivitis means inflammation of the gingiva (gums).

At one time, a physician's diagnosis typically included both the symptoms and the apparent cause of a disease. Unfortunately, that has changed, and the diagnosis of an -itis disease (and most other diseases as well) is now often nothing more than a description of symptoms. Dermatitis, an inflammation of the skin, can have many causes, including allergies, infections, a toxic reaction to a chemical, or abrasion.

In the case of coronary artery disease, something inflames the blood vessel walls, triggering a cascade of events. That "something" might be a corrosive protein by-product called homocysteine, a low-grade infection, or oxidized cholesterol, all of which increase the risk of developing heart disease. (This relationship between inflammation and cardiovascular disease will be discussed in depth in later chapters.) In response, white blood cells migrate to artery walls, where they release free radicals, fuel inflammation, and exacerbate the damage. The most accurate predictor of whether you will have a heart attack is not your cholesterol, triglyceride, or blood sugar level. Rather, it is a high blood level of C-reactive protein, an indicator of your body's overall inflammation.

—m—

Common Inflammatory Diseases and Disorders

Inflammation is a symptom of virtually every disease process, and it often makes the condition worse. These are some examples of common disorders that involve inflammation:

Arthritis
    Osteoarthritis
    Rheumatoid arthritis
Injuries
    Athletic: tendinitis, bursitis, muscle strains, and bruises
    Cuts, broken bones, bruises, surgery
Infections
    Colds, flus, otitis media, hepatitis C, HIV, parasites
    Vague low-grade infections, Epstein-Barr disease
Allergies/autoimmune problems
    Pollen and other inhalant allergies (rhinitis, nonallergic rhinitis)
    Food allergies
    Celiac disease (gluten intolerance)
    Lupus erythematosus
Pulmonary
    Asthma
    Chronic obstructive pulmonary disease
    Bronchitis
Cardiovascular
    Coronary artery disease, myocarditis, hypertension
    Stroke
    Phlebitis, varicose veins
Cancer
    Various types, including gastric, lung, breast, and prostate
Neurological
    Alzheimer's disease
Skin
    Sunburn (erythema)
    Eczema and dermatitis
    Psoriasis
Dental
    Gingivitis
    Periodontitis

Eye
  Conjunctivitis
  Uveitis
Digestive tract
  Gastritis, ulcers
  Crohn's disease
  Ulcerative colitis
  Inflammatory bowel disease
  Diverticulitis
Miscellaneous
  Sinusitis
  Multiple sclerosis
  Obesity
  Diabetes

—⁓—

The Prevalence of Inflammation

One way to look at the prevalence of inflammatory diseases is to track the sales (and, by implication, the use) of anti-inflammatory drugs such as aspirin, ibuprofen, naproxen sodium, and Cox-2 inhibitors. Each year more than 30 billion tablets of nonsteroidal anti-inflammatory drugs (NSAIDs) are sold over the counter in the United States—more than one hundred for every man, woman, and child. In addition, doctors write 70 million prescriptions for even stronger NSAIDs. Although some NSAIDs are often used to treat headaches (which may be caused by inflammation), these numbers reflect an enormous dependency on anti-inflammatory drugs.

Indeed, one piece of evidence that coronary artery disease and Alzheimer's disease are inflammatory diseases is the fact that both may be prevented with certain anti-inflammatory drugs. Aspirin reduces the risk of suffering a heart attack, and ibuprofen (the active ingredient in Advil) appears to reduce the risk of developing Alzheimer's disease. Unfortunately, serious and sometimes life-threatening side effects are common from both drugs, which make them undesirable approaches to prevention or treatment.

None of these drugs treats the underlying causes of inflammation. At best, they provide short-term relief. Worse, some NSAIDs hasten the breakdown of joint cartilage, aggravating the damage and speeding the progression of osteoarthritis. You will learn more about the dangers of anti-inflammatory drugs in chapter 5.

CHAPTER 2

Your Inflammation Triggers

Georgia: Allergies and Sinusitis

Georgia had suffered from chronic sinusitis, an inflammation or infection of the air spaces near the nose, since she was twelve and developed asthma at age forty-one. She was also allergic to dust, grasses, smoke, perfumes, wool, and some cosmetics. Within a few years of her asthma diagnosis, Georgia was taking a variety of prescription drugs: oral and nasal, a bronchodilator, antibiotics, and other medications. She began to feel addicted to her asthma drugs and was afraid to be without them.

Her asthma was related to and aggravated by the sinus problems, and Georgia found herself taking increasingly stronger medications. She was also having frequent and severe headaches. At age fifty-two, she consulted holistic physician Robert S. Ivker, D.O., of Denver, Colorado, the author of several books, including *Sinus Survival*, *Asthma Survival*, and *Headache Survival*.

Ivker recommended a number of nutritional supplements, including vitamins E and C, beta-carotene, selenium, zinc, and an overall multivitamin, as well as an herbal echinacea and goldenseal combination. He also treated Georgia for a Candida infection and recommended that she purchase a negative-ion generator to improve the air quality in her home. These changes were combined with a tapering off of some of her medications and the beginning of a gradual exercise program, with Georgia riding a stationary bicycle and walking.

Two months after Georgia's first visit to Ivker, she had a new vitality and higher energy levels. She had also lost five pounds. Over the next year or so, she was able to stop using all of her medications. Recognizing the role of emotion in illness, Ivker asked Georgia to focus on strengthening her family relationships. Today, with her newfound health, Georgia and her husband are planning for an active retirement.

Inflammation Triggers

Nearly everyone confuses the *causes* of inflammation with its *triggers*. For example, pollen does not by itself cause an inflammatory response. Rather it triggers an inflammatory response in susceptible individuals. The causes of inflammation are often related to dietary imbalances or deficiencies, which prime the immune system for a powerful and chronic inflammatory reaction.

Inflammation triggers are the events that precipitate a specific inflammatory response *after* the body is already primed for an overreaction. Although it is not the same as correcting the causes of inflammation, it is essential to avoid events that trigger inflammation. Doing so helps settle down an agitated immune system.

First, try to reduce your exposure to inflammation triggers. For example, if you have food allergies, make a point of avoiding troublesome foods. Similarly, if you are a weekend-warrior athlete who frequently gets injured, it might be good to take up a more moderate and regular physical activity, such as swimming or walking. Repeated injuries keep revving up the body's inflammatory response.

Second, it is important to dampen the immune response to unavoidable triggers (e.g., seasonal pollen allergies). And third, it would be ideal to normalize the immune response to inflammation triggers. The second and third approaches rely chiefly on your making dietary changes and taking nutritional supplements, and these approaches are discussed in depth in later chapters.

For now, there are eight general categories of inflammatory triggers to understand.

1. Age-Related Wear and Tear: What Is Your *Biological* Age?

Every living creature ages, and age is characterized by less biological efficiency and an accelerated breakdown of tissue and normal biochemical processes. When tissues break down, white blood cells are mobilized to clean up, in a manner of speaking, the biological dust. The aging process occurs at individual rates of speed and is influenced by a variety of factors, including genetics, diet, frequency of infections, stress, and overall lifestyle. Of particular interest, levels of the body's key pro-inflammatory substances generally increase with age. This rise may be due to age-related tissue breakdown—and the immune system's response to it—or perhaps to the long-term effect of eating a pro-inflammatory diet.

Although most of us think of our age chronologically, our biological age is actually far more important. Chronological age refers to how many years old a person is, whereas biological age assesses age in terms of physical and mental performance. Many people in their seventies and eighties have more vigor and better health than do people half their age. Some researchers have noted that healthy centenarians are not simply healthy old people. They are often healthier than younger seniors and in many ways on a par with people in their forties.

One way to maintain a lower biological age is to reduce tissue breakdown and the inflammation it stimulates. In a general way, diets rich in vegetables and fruits provide large quantities of antioxidants, such as vitamin C, carotenoids, and flavonoids. These antioxidants neutralize damaging free radicals. For example, people who eat large amounts of antioxidant-rich vegetables develop fewer wrinkles and look younger. As another example, many people take glucosamine sulfate supplements, which help them maintain "younger" joints and reduce the pain of osteoarthritis. Both glucosamine and chondroitin also have anti-inflammatory benefits.

2. Physical Injuries

Physical injuries can accelerate the aging of specific tissues, such as joints, muscles, and bone. Many such injuries, such as falling and breaking a bone or musculoskeletal athletic injuries, can become the source of painful and debilitating lifelong health problems. Former heavyweight boxing champion Muhammad Ali, who was physically and mentally agile as a young man, developed Parkinson's disease as a consequence of cumulative brain damage in the ring. Injuries become sources of chronic inflammation and pain because they are initially serious, repeated, do not heal properly, or promote sustained low-grade inflammation in the damaged tissues.

To minimize your chances of suffering a physical injury, it is important to be aware of your immediate environment and to avoid reckless behavior. For example, drive defensively and watch where you step. As you reach middle and old age, it may be better to adopt low-impact physical activities, such as swimming or walking.

3. Infections

Researchers reported in the journal *Circulation* that repeated infections greatly increased a person's risk of dying from coronary artery disease. Literally, the more infections people experienced, the more likely they were to develop and die from heart disease. It wasn't that the bacteria and the viruses were directly infecting the heart. More likely, repeated infections maintained higher activity in immune cells, elevated CRP levels, and damaged arteries.

Infections turn on the body's most powerful inflammatory responses, and sometimes the body ends up fighting itself. For example, a person who catches one cold after another suffers through a state of near-chronic inflammation with periodic peaks of inflammation, which slowly but surely attack and break down the entire body.

It is possible, nutritionally, to boost the *efficiency* of the immune system's response to infections. Vitamins C and E and a nutritional supplement called N-acetylcysteine (NAC) can greatly reduce the inflammatory symptoms of infections.

4. Environmental Stresses

Many common environmental stresses can also cause acute and chronic inflammatory responses. For example, tobacco smoke and other forms of air pollution irritate the lungs and activate large numbers of white blood cells, which contribute to further damage.

Cold air and exercise trigger severe asthma attacks in many people. The immune system of a person with asthma misreads the physiological changes triggered by cold air and exercise and overreacts to them. People with asthma are known to have abnormally high levels of free radicals, which promote inflammation, but these can be reduced with such antioxidants as vitamin C, lycopene, and beta-carotene.

5. Allergies and Food Sensitivities

Pollen allergies, such as to ragweed, are common and have been increasing in prevalence. The most common allergenic pollens are from grasses, trees, and weeds, with sensitive people reacting when these plants release pollen into the air. Many people are also allergic to molds and dust. Their symptoms are collectively referred to as allergic rhinitis. About 15 percent of the North American population suffers from seasonal allergic rhinitis, and millions more people experience nonallergic rhinitis—basically, nasal congestion or a runny nose unrelated to inhaled allergens.

People with pollen allergies have a higher than average risk of developing asthma, and people with multiple pollen (and other inhalant) allergies have an even greater chance. According to the National Heart, Lung, and Blood Institute, the incidence of asthma increased by 75 percent between 1980 and 1994. These numbers have continued to climb, and now more than 22 million Americans have asthma (an increase of 5 million since 2002 alone). Its prevalence has also increased in other nations where the condition was once rare.

Researchers have for many years tried to identify a single environmental cause to account for the sharp rise in the incidence of asthma. Some of the suspects include dust mites, cockroach feces, and overzealous hygiene (which prevents normal programming of the immune system). It is very unlikely that any single cause can be blamed. Rather, the greater prevalence of asthma (as well as of pollen allergies) is likely the result of multiple factors, including the biochemical consequences of significant dietary changes, indoor air pollution (from the outgassing of synthetic carpets, plastics, and glues used in construction materials), and allergic parents giving birth to allergic and more asthmatically susceptible children.

Food sensitivities are allergylike reactions. Some common allergies, such as to peanuts or shrimp, raise levels of IgE (immunoglobulin E), the conventional marker of an allergy. Beyond this, the topic of food allergies has often been charged with controversy because it has been difficult to identify a specific immune sign of a reaction. In recent years, however, some physicians have found that many food allergens raise levels of IgG, which, like IgE, triggers a cascade of events that alters physical health and cognitive functioning. Because blood tests may not always identify a specific immune reaction, you may have to rely on symptoms in response to specific foods.

Nutritionally oriented physicians recommend strict avoidance of food allergens, and they often suggest that patients follow a "rotation diet" to reduce the likelihood of new food allergies developing. A rotation diet prohibits eating the same food or food from the same family (such as dairy) more often than once every four days. Sometimes allergic reactivity will diminish after several months of avoiding problematic foods.

Maureen: Drugs Didn't Work

Maureen, a fifty-seven-year-old woman, had chronic but mild and manageable muscle and joint pains. She rarely ate tomatoes until her neighbor shared with her a bumper crop of tomatoes and eggplants, foods that are members of the nightshade plant family.

She soon began to experience a significant increase in joint pain, which was not relieved by anti-inflammatory medications. When Maureen related her health history to Hunter Yost, M.D., of Tucson, Arizona, he immediately recognized the likely cause of her increased pain: she is one of those people who are nightshade-sensitive.

Dr. Yost asked her to immediately stop eating all nightshades, a food category that also includes red and green peppers and potatoes. Within one week of eliminating these foods, Maureen had a significant decrease in joint pain, although her muscle pain did persist.

6. Dietary Imbalances and Deficiencies

Many dietary factors besides food allergies can set the stage for chronic inflammation. Chief among them is an unbalanced intake of certain dietary fats, leading to a functional deficiency of some of them. Two families of dietary fats, known as the omega-3s and the omega-6s, provide the biochemical building blocks for the body's anti-inflammatory and pro-inflammatory compounds. Most processed and packaged foods—that is, those sold in boxes, cans, jars, and bottles—contain negligible amounts of the anti-inflammatory omega-3 fats. In contrast, they contain abnormally large amounts of pro-inflammatory omega-6 fats. The richest sources of omega-3 fats are coldwater fish, such as salmon and sardines, whereas most omega-6 fats come from safflower, peanut, and corn oils. I'll explain more about these fats in chapters 3 and 8.

In addition to unbalanced fat intake, nine out of ten Americans don't eat sufficient amounts of vegetables and fruits, which are rich in antioxidants, anti-inflammatory vitamins, and other nutrients. Vitamins C and E, as well as flavonoids (a family of nutrients that adds color to vegetables and fruits), have potent anti-inflammatory benefits.

These low levels of omega-3 fats and antioxidants promote abnormal inflammatory responses. Many cases of inflammatory disorders, such as arthritis and allergies, have been resolved simply by taking omega-3 fish oil and antioxidant supplements.

7. "Leaky Gut" Syndrome

Many nutritionally oriented physicians diagnose and treat "leaky gut" syndrome. The condition is characterized by a highly permeable digestive tract that enables undigested or partially digested food proteins to directly enter the bloodstream, where they prompt an inflammatory response.

Leaky gut syndrome is often the consequence of dysbiosis, or a catastrophic disruption in the beneficial bacteria that normally inhabit the digestive tract. What causes dysbiosis? It can be the result of poor dietary habits, chlorine in drinking water, stomach flu, or food poisoning. But more often than not, it can be traced to the use of oral antibiotics. Dysbiosis is why many people develop diarrhea after taking antibiotics, and some people continue to suffer the consequences of antibiotics for years after they cease taking the drugs.

Antibiotics tend to be indiscriminate and typically kill off large numbers of beneficial bacteria, along with those that cause disease. By destroying beneficial bacteria, antibiotics create a microbial vacuum that enables opportunistic disease-causing microorganisms, such as *C. albicans* and *Clostridium difficile*, to take root and cause secondary infections. In particular, *C. albicans* (yeast) infections can be either localized (such as in the vagina) or systemic (causing a variety of difficult-to-diagnose symptoms).

The importance of healthy gut bacteria cannot be understated. Normally, these bacteria make small amounts of certain vitamins and help us digest food, but they are also important regulators of immunity and inflammation. (In fact, you have about ten times more bacteria in your gut than cells in your entire body.) Recent research has shown that imbalances in gut bacteria predispose at least some people toward weight gain. Perhaps more worrisome, the use of antibiotics to treat ear infections in infants and toddlers may fundamentally alter their gut bacteria and inflammatory responses, making them more susceptible to obesity, allergies, and asthma as they grow into children and adults.

8. Prediabetes, Diabetes, and Overweight

People with prediabetes, diabetes, or excess weight tend to have elevated levels of C-reactive protein or other indicators of inflammation. Prediabetes and type 2 diabetes are almost always intertwined with overweight and obesity, specifically abdominal obesity (that is, a big belly). So, what causes the higher level of inflammation in people with these health problems?

First, a high intake of dietary sugars (such as sucrose and high-fructose corn syrup) and refined grains (white bread, muffins, pasta) elevates blood sugar and insulin levels. Insulin increases the secretion of C-reactive protein (CRP), while high blood sugar intensifies the production of free radicals, molecules that help promote and sustain inflammation.

Second, rather than simply hanging around the waist, fat cells are biologically active. They secrete inflammation-promoting compounds, such as interleukin-6 and CRP. Interleukin-6 is one of the most powerful inflammatory molecules in the body, and CRP is a by-product of it. Both substances help produce what researchers call an inflammatory cascade. Think of the cascade as being somewhat similar to a falling row of dominoes, except that the cascade results in more and more inflammation-causing changes. As part of this cascade, white blood cells migrate to the spaces between fat cells, and the white blood cells secrete their own interleukin-6 and CRP and further fuel the inflammatory cascade. These high levels of interleukin-6, CRP, and free radicals amount to biochemical triggers, waiting for the slightest provocation to further fuel the fires of inflammation.

Cytokines also increase the risk of developing insulin resistance, which is the cornerstone of prediabetes and type 2 diabetes. (See my book *Stop Prediabetes Now* for an in-depth discussion of these issues.) Insulin resistance is characterized by high levels of the hormone insulin, but cells resist its normal glucose-regulating effects. Based on an article in the March–April 2008 issue of *Molecular Medicine*, CRP and many of the other pro-inflammatory cytokines interfere with the normal activity of insulin. This essentially means that prediabetes (which in some form affects an estimated 100 million Americans) can stimulate inflammation, while inflammation also increases the risk of prediabetes, type 2 diabetes, and overweight. In fact, pro-inflammatory cytokines can cause insulin resistance even in the absence of overweight.

The next chapter explains what happens during an inflammatory reaction, how the body makes powerful inflammation-producing substances from foods, and why many foods make us overreact to inflammation triggers.

CHAPTER 3

The Dietary Causes
of Inflammation

If injuries, infections, pollens, and other physical insults merely trigger inflammatory reactions, the obvious question is: What makes a normal process go out of control?

The answer lies in the foods we eat. If you eat the typical North American (or Western) diet, loaded with convenience and fast foods, you likely consume too many of the nutrients that promote inflammation—and not enough of those that reduce inflammation. This imbalance results in large part from massive changes to our food supply over the last fifty years or so. During this time, highly processed pro-inflammatory foods have largely replaced anti-inflammatory fresh and natural foods. This has primed our bodies to develop chronic, excessive, and self-destructive levels of inflammation.

How do foods affect inflammation? Nutrients provide the building blocks of your body and, of particular importance, your immune system, which regulates inflammation. Your immune system consists of hundreds of specialized types of cells and molecules that constantly monitor your body for anything "foreign" or unusual. To envision this, it might help to picture how a taut, silken web alerts its resident spider to the presence of an insect. When a fly touches some threads in the web, the resulting vibrations are transmitted and amplified throughout the web. These vibrations alert the spider, which moves in for the kill.

The cells of the immune system operate much like the interlocking filaments of the spider web. An immune cell senses the presence of an intruder (such as infectious bacteria or some other material—for example, a damaged or dead cell) that does not belong in the body. An immune cell quickly shares information about the peculiarity with other immune cells. Together, they coordinate a response and, if the immune system is working properly, dispose of the foreign material.

You might wonder whether a powerful immune response is really necessary, but there is a biological rationale for it. Historically, infections have been the leading cause of human deaths. Even today, infections remain the third leading cause of death in the United States and the leading cause worldwide. A strong immune response has always given us a fighting chance against infections. Intense inflammatory responses are inappropriate, however, when they target healthy tissues or harmless pollens, or when the body lacks normal switches to turn off inflammation.

Barbara: Inflammation, Rheumatoid Arthritis, and Asthma

At age forty-one, Barbara had suffered with rheumatoid arthritis and asthma for years and was taking half a dozen prescription drugs, which barely kept her symptoms in check. Then Barbara's physician started her on the hormone prednisone. After seven months on the drug, she had gained 100 pounds—she was carrying 251 pounds on her 5'2" frame—and also developed the "moon face" that is characteristic of prednisone users. The cure was worse than the disease.

As a last-ditch effort, she went to a nutritionally oriented medical center in Wichita, Kansas. There, Hugh D. Riordan, M.D., and Ronald E. Hunninghake, M.D., found Barbara to be low in two essential "good" fats that are natural anti-inflammatory nutrients, as well as low in vitamins C and E and other nutrients. Lab tests also determined that Barbara had several allergylike food and chemical sensitivities, which helped fuel her overactive immune system and runaway inflammation.

The prescription was remarkably simple. Drs. Riordan and Hunninghake recommended that Barbara eat a more wholesome diet, avoid the foods and the chemicals she was sensitive to, and take fish oil supplements (which contain the good fats) and vitamins. Nine months later, her asthma was completely gone, her arthritic symptoms were so mild that she reduced her prednisone to less than one-thousandth of the dose she had been taking—from 40 mg daily to 1 mg per month—and she was able to stop taking all of the other medications. Barbara had also lost seventy pounds, and her outlook toward life changed as well. She was now energetic, upbeat, and outgoing.

Pro- and Anti-Inflammatory Counterbalances

With all the bad news we hear about fats, it may surprise you to read that some types of fats form the foundation of the body's pro- and anti-inflammatory compounds. Contrary to what you may have heard, fats (also known as fatty acids) are not inherently bad for your health. Many fats are as essential for good health as proteins, carbohydrates, vitamins, and minerals are. Pro- and anti-inflammatory fats should serve as counterbalances to each other. Chronic inflammation can develop when there is a sharp imbalance in the types of fats you consume.

To understand how some fats increase or decrease inflammation, it helps to see them (and other pro- and anti-inflammatory substances) in simple terms, such as "matches" or "firefighters." Chronic inflammation often results from too many dietary matches. By making greater use of dietary firefighters, however, you can restore a balance that prevents or even reverses chronic inflammation.

Pro-Inflammatory Fats

Two specific types of fats, as well as free radicals, prime our bodies for inflammation. Here is a brief description of them.

- The *omega-6* family of fatty acids supplies the building blocks of a variety of powerful pro-inflammatory substances. The omega-6 fatty acids are commonly found as *linoleic acid*, most often in vegetable oils such as corn, safflower, peanut, cottonseed, and soy oils, as well as in processed and packaged foods containing these oils. Arachidonic acid, one of the omega-6 fatty acids, stimulates the body's production of many other inflammation-causing chemicals, such as prostaglandin E_2.
- *Trans-fatty acids* are hidden in products that contain "partially hydrogenated vegetable oils," such as salad dressings, breakfast bars, shortening, nondairy creamers, stick margarines, and many baked items such as cakes and cookies. Omega-6 vegetable oils

are bad enough in themselves, but hydrogenation gives them many of the characteristics of saturated fats. Trans-fatty acids do much of their damage by interfering with the body's handling of anti-inflammatory fats, specifically the omega-3 fatty acids.

Anti-Inflammatory Fats

Three specific types of fats, as well as antioxidant nutrients, help control inflammation. Here is a brief overview of them.

- The *omega-3* family of fatty acids supplies the building blocks of a variety of powerful anti-inflammatory substances. The parent fat of the omega-3s, *alpha-linolenic acid*, is found in dark green leafy vegetables and flaxseed. More potent omega-3s, especially EPA (eicosapentaenoic acid), are found in coldwater fish such as salmon and herring. Basically, the omega-3s encourage the body's production of inflammation-suppressing compounds, such as prostaglandin E_3. The omega-3s help remind the body to turn inflammatory reactions off when they are no longer needed.
- *GLA (gamma-linolenic acid)* is technically an omega-6 fatty acid, but it behaves more like an anti-inflammatory omega-3. The body converts GLA to prostaglandin E_1, which is anti-inflammatory. It enhances the inflammation-suppressing effect of omega-3s.
- The *omega-9* family of fatty acids works with the omega-3s as anti-inflammatory compounds. Omega-9s are found in olive oil, avocados, macadamia nuts, and macadamia nut oil.

—◊◊◊—

Rev Up Your Body's Natural Anti-Inflammatories

One of the best anti-inflammatory supplements on the market combines several of my top nutrients—omega-3 fish oils, gamma-linolenic acid, vitamin D, and vitamin E. Inflammation Balance was developed by Carlson Laboratories and is sold through many health and natural food stores. You can take one to three capsules daily for either chronic aches and pains or recent injuries. (For more information, visit carlsonlabs.com, or call 1-800-323-4141.)

—◊◊◊—

The Pro-Inflammatory Pathway . . .
But Not Always

The omega-6 fatty acids are one of two families of polyunsaturated fats and oils. *Linoleic acid*, found in most cooking oils, is the "parent molecule" of all other omega-6 fatty acids. It is essential for health, but the modern diet provides far too much of it, creating a biochemical setting that encourages chronic inflammation. The widespread modern use of vegetable cooking oils (chiefly, corn, safflower, soybean, and peanut oils) is a principal reason for the increasing prevalence of inflammatory disorders.

By itself, linoleic acid does not have much biological activity, but its biochemical "children" do. One line of descent (or biochemical pathway) from linoleic acid leads to the production of *arachidonic acid*, which is the true hub of the omega-6s' pro-inflammatory effects. Diets high in linoleic acid increase the production of arachidonic acid, and corn-fed meats are particularly rich in arachidonic acid. Of all the meats, pork is especially high in arachidonic acid, possibly because pigs (like people) will eat almost anything. Through a number of steps, arachidonic acid is converted to prostaglandin E_2 and leukotriene B_4, both powerful promoters of inflammation. The conversion of arachidonic acid to prostaglandin E_2 is strongly influenced by interleukin-6 and CRP.

Although the omega-6s are widely regarded as being pro-inflammatory, some members of the family exert powerful anti-inflammatory benefits—in effect, they are natural checks and balances to the pro-inflammatory power of arachidonic acid. Chief among these is *gamma-linolenic acid* (to be discussed more in chapter 8), which is converted to dihomo-gamma-linolenic acid and then to anti-inflammatory prostaglandin E_1. (Refer to the illustration on page 40 to see the actual steps.)

Furthermore, some arachidonic acid itself can be converted to a family of anti-inflammatory molecules called lipoxins. The production of lipoxins requires the presence of aspirin, but you probably don't have to take aspirin (if you would rather avoid all drugs). Culinary herbs and spices are rich in salicylic acid, the "natural" form of aspirin, and vegetables and fruits also contain appreciable amounts of salicylic acid.

By the way, if you are a little confused about pro- and anti-inflammatory prostaglandins and leukotrienes, here's an easy way to keep them straight: most of those with an even number are pro-inflammatory, whereas those with an odd number are anti-inflammatory.

—⁓—

What Are Cytokines?

Cytokines (pronounced sight-o-kines) are a family of cell-communication molecules. This means they are involved in how the body's cells talk with one another. Cytokines play a particularly important role in regulating the immune system, which revs up inflammation to fight infections and also to initiate the healing process. In people who have chronic inflammation, levels of several cytokines may be elevated. These include interleukin-6 (IL-6) and its by-product C-reactive protein (CRP), as well as tumor necrosis factor alpha (TNF-a), interleukin-1 beta (IL-1b), and leukotriene B_4 (LTB4). CRP is the easiest and least expensive to measure, and doctors tend to use the high-sensitivity CRP test (hsCRP) to gauge inflammation.

—⁓—

The Anti-Inflammatory Pathway

Like the omega-6s, the omega-3 fatty acids are a family of polyunsaturated fats and oils. Both families of fatty acids exist as separate, but parallel, biochemical pathways.

Alpha-linolenic acid is the parent molecule of many members of the body's anti-inflammatory omega-3 fatty acid family. The omega-3s, however, are less active biologically than are the omega-6 fatty acids. As a result, you have to make an extra effort to consume foods or supplements rich in omega-3 fatty acids to make up for their weaker activity.

Under ideal circumstances, alpha-linolenic acid, which is abundant in leafy green vegetables and flaxseed, gets converted to stearidonic acid (found in echium oil, which may soon be available as a supplement). Stearidonic acid is readily converted through a couple of steps to eicosapentaenoic acid (EPA), which is eventually turned into docosahexaenoic acid (DHA) (see the illustration on page 41). Fish oil supplements have the advantage of being rich in EPA and DHA, leapfrogging the many steps needed to make EPA and DHA in the body.

EPA is the principal hub of the body's anti-inflammatory compounds. Through the action of two specialized enzymes, EPA gets made into anti-inflammatory prostaglandin E_3 and leukotriene B_5. In addition, some EPA and DHA gets converted to a recently discovered group of anti-inflammatory compounds—resolvins, neuroprotectins, and lipoxins.

In our evolutionary and dietary past, people consumed roughly equal amounts of omega-6 and omega-3 fats. Today, because of the extensive use of processed oils in convenience and fast foods, people now consume twenty to thirty times more omega-6s relative to omega-3s. Worse, these are low-quality omega-6s, rich in linoleic acid and arachidonic acid. This lopsided intake of omega-6s smothers the already minuscule dietary amounts of alpha-linolenic acid, EPA, DHA, and GLA, further suppressing the body's ability to control inflammation.

It's important to mention the synergism among EPA, DHA, and GLA. They work far better together—that is, EPA and DHA combined with GLA—than separately. By increasing the body's production of anti-inflammatory prostaglandin E_1 and prostaglandin E_3, these nutritional substances counteract the pro-inflammatory effects of prostaglandin E_2. This very combination of nutrients has been used with great success to enhance recovery among athletes on the Danish Olympic teams. In the same vein, the German Weight Lifting Federation and the German weight-lifting team have used a high-EPA form of fish oil to ease muscle soreness.

The Amazing Resolvins, Protectins, and Lipoxins

These days, it's uncommon for researchers to discover new and significant nutrient-related compounds. Yet over the last few years, Charles N. Serhan, Ph.D., and his colleagues at the Harvard Medical School have discovered and have been investigating several new families of anti-inflammatory compounds that are by-products of dietary fatty acids. Among them are resolvins, protectins (neuroprotectins), and lipoxins. Although the body makes these substances in very tiny quantities, they are among the most powerful of all anti-inflammatory chemicals.

Resolvins, protectins, and neuroprotectins are made in the omega-3 pathway. The name *resolvin* reflects the substance's role in resolving inflammation. The resolvin E family is a by-product of EPA, whereas the resolvin D family is made from DHA. Similarly, the term *protectin* suggests a protective role, and protectin D_1 is derived from DHA.

In experiments, Serhan showed that resolvin E_1 inhibited the activation and movement of immune cells, a change that would diminish inflammation. It also reduced skin inflammation and reversed periodontal disease in laboratory animals. Resolvin E_1 works in part by turning off production of nuclear factor kappa beta, a protein that activates inflammation-promoting genes. Meanwhile, protectins protect against

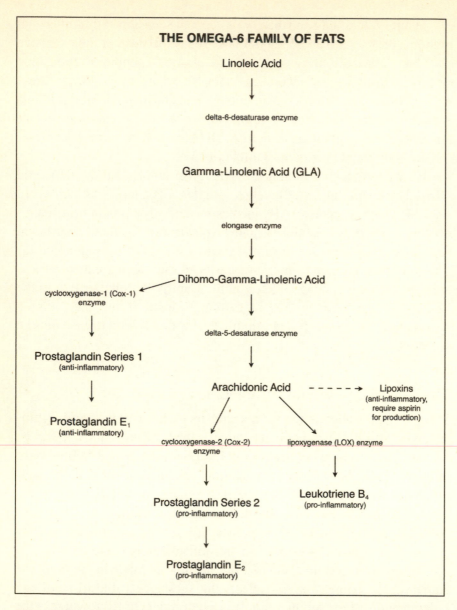

THE OMEGA-6 FAMILY OF FATS

Linoleic Acid

↓

delta-6-desaturase enzyme

↓

Gamma-Linolenic Acid (GLA)

↓

elongase enzyme

↓

Dihomo-Gamma-Linolenic Acid

cyclooxygenase-1 (Cox-1) enzyme ← | ↓ delta-5-desaturase enzyme

Prostaglandin Series 1 (anti-inflammatory)

↓

Prostaglandin E_1 (anti-inflammatory)

Arachidonic Acid – – – → Lipoxins (anti-inflammatory, require aspirin for production)

cyclooxygenase-2 (Cox-2) enzyme   lipoxygenase (LOX) enzyme

Prostaglandin Series 2 (pro-inflammatory)   Leukotriene B_4 (pro-inflammatory)

↓

Prostaglandin E_2 (pro-inflammatory)

Although the omega-6 fatty acid pathway is commonly considered pro-inflammatory, much of it can be anti-inflammatory. The parent molecule is linoleic acid, found in corn, soybean, safflower, and peanut oils. It is converted to gamma-linolenic acid by way of the delta-6-desaturase enzyme. The hub of the pro-inflammatory pathway is arachidonic acid, which is converted to pro-inflammatory prostaglandins (for example, prostaglandin E_2) and leuko-trienes (such as leukotriene B_4). In the presence of aspirin, however, some arachidonic acid can be converted to anti-inflammatory lipoxins. A stronger anti-inflammatory pathway is mediated by the Cox-1 enzyme, which converts dihomo-gamma-linolenic acid to anti-inflammatory prostaglandins (such as prostaglandin E_1). Large amounts of linoleic acid and corn-fed meats in the diet increase arachidonic acid levels. In addition, trans fats and alcohol inhibit the activity of the delta-6-desaturase enzyme.

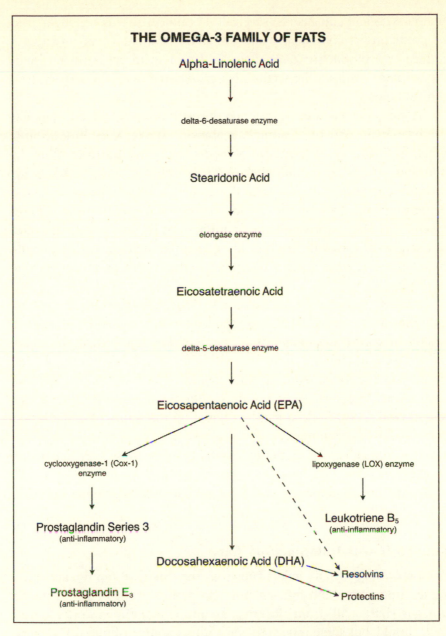

THE OMEGA-3 FAMILY OF FATS

Alpha-Linolenic Acid

↓

delta-6-desaturase enzyme

↓

Stearidonic Acid

↓

elongase enzyme

↓

Eicosatetraenoic Acid

↓

delta-5-desaturase enzyme

↓

Eicosapentaenoic Acid (EPA)

cyclooxygenase-1 (Cox-1)
enzyme

lipoxygenase (LOX) enzyme

Leukotriene B₅
(anti-inflammatory)

Prostaglandin Series 3
(anti-inflammatory)

Docosahexaenoic Acid (DHA)

Resolvins

Prostaglandin E₃
(anti-inflammatory)

Protectins

The omega-3 pathway is anti-inflammatory and dampens the pro-inflammatory aspects of the omega-6 pathway. Linolenic acid, found in leafy green vegetables and flaxseed, is the parent molecule of the omega-3s. EPA is the hub of the omega-3s' anti-inflammatory activities, and it is converted to anti-inflammatory prostaglandins (such as prostaglandin E_1) and leukotrienes (such as leukotriene B_5). EPA and DHA also lead to the production of small amounts of very potent anti-inflammatory compounds called resolvins and protectins. Trans fats and alcohol interfere with the activity of the delta-6-desaturase enzyme, which inhibits the early steps in the omega-3 pathway. Fish oil supplements have the advantage of being rich in EPA and DHA and therefore bypass those steps.

41

brain toxins and enhance the survival of brain cells. This beneficial role of protectins is consistent with how DHA (the source of protectins) reduces the production of beta-amyloid protein (a causative factor in Alzheimer's disease). Protectins also protect the eye's retina from free radical damage.

Aspirin increases the production of resolvins and protectins, which might explain part of the drug's analgesic effects. Very little aspirin (acetylsalicylic acid) is needed to boost resolvins and protectins. In addition, people can produce their own salicylic acid from benzoic acid, another compound that is naturally found in vegetables and fruits, according to a 2008 article in the *Journal of Agricultural and Food Chemistry*. Not surprisingly, the combination of fish, vegetables, and kitchen herbs forms the heart of my anti-inflammatory dietary recommendations—and is another testament to the health-promoting power of foods.

Interestingly enough, arachidonic acid (the hub of pro-inflammatory activities in the omega-6 pathway) can lead to the production of another family of potent anti-inflammatory compounds, lipoxins. In this case, aspirin (or salicylic acid) is necessary for the conversion of some arachidonic acid to lipoxins. Animal and cell studies have shown that lipoxins function as "braking signals" to reduce inflammation and swelling and to lessen pain. They work in part by regulating the influx of white blood cells to sites of inflammation.

Unfortunately, you can't buy resolvins, protectins, and lipoxins as supplements. You can, however, certainly increase your body's production of them with supplements of omega-3 fish oils and gamma-linolenic acid.

Omega-9 Anti-Inflammatory Fats

Another group of fatty acids, known as the omega-9 family, also possesses impressive anti-inflammatory properties. Your body can make omega-9 fatty acids from other fats, assuming that things work the way they should, but some foods provide a direct source of them. The basic building block of the omega-9 fatty acids is oleic acid, a monounsaturated fat found abundantly in olive oil, macadamia nuts, and avocados.

Many studies have found that diets rich in olive oil reduce the risk or severity of inflammatory diseases such as coronary artery disease and rheumatoid arthritis. In general, the omega-9 family is synergistic with the anti-inflammatory omega-3 family.

Skewing the Balance with Trans Fats

The widespread use of trans fats, found in "partially hydrogenated" vegetable oils, has further compromised our bodies' ability to control inflammation and inflammation-related health problems.

Beginning in the 1960s, public health officials urged people to consume more polyunsaturated fats, particularly the omega-6 variety, and to eat fewer saturated fats. Food makers increasingly used hydrogenated vegetable oils, which provide the texture of saturated fats, such as butter. Until the early 1990s, almost everyone thought hydrogenated oils were safe. It turns out that they are anything but safe—and there is no safe amount of them.

The first sign that trans fats might be troublesome came in a study published in 1982 in the *Proceedings of the National Academy of Sciences*. In that study, researchers reported that trans fats interfered with the activity of an enzyme, delta-6-desaturase (D6D). This would have been nothing more than a bit of arcane biochemistry were it not for the fact that D6D plays two pivotal roles: first in converting linoleic acid to gamma-linolenic acid, and second in converting alpha-linolenic acid to stearidonic acid. Essentially, trans fats put the brakes on the first step in both the omega-6 and the omega-3 pathways. (To see the role of D6D in the omega-6 and omega-3 pathways, refer to the figures on pages 40–41.)

Public health experts see the consumption of foods with trans fats as a risk factor for developing coronary heart disease. The reason is that trans fats raise levels of the "bad" low-density lipoprotein (LDL) form of cholesterol and lower levels of the "good" high-density lipoprotein (HDL) form of cholesterol.

The other negative health effects of trans fats appear to be far greater, though. By inhibiting D6D, trans fats fundamentally alter how the body processes fats. One consequence is that trans fats increase the formation of belly fat, which is worse than any other type of body fat for boosting the risk of diabetes and heart disease. Trans fats also increase insulin resistance, the hallmark of prediabetes and type 2 diabetes.

It took until 2006 for the Food and Drug Administration to require food companies to list trans fats in the Nutrition Facts boxes on food packages. But the FDA gave food companies a loophole. Food makers could list the amount of trans fats as zero if the food contained less than one-half (0.5) gram of trans fats *per serving*. In other words, 0.49 gram of trans fats could be listed as zero. With official serving sizes routinely understated, it's easy to consume two or three servings of a particular food and thus to consume substantial amounts of trans fats.

Interesterified Fats—Worse Than Trans Fats

In 2007, the giant food company Archer Daniels Midland began to market "interesterified vegetable oils" as a replacement for trans fats. It turns out that interesterified oils are actually worse than trans fats! Interesterified oils raise LDL and lower HDL, just as trans fats do. But a study of people who consumed interesterified fats found that these also increased blood sugar by 20 to 40 percent in just one month—in effect, putting people on the fast track to developing diabetes.

Although interesterified fats are marketed as an industry-friendly replacement for trans fats, some varieties actually contain trans fats. The advantage of this shell game for the junk-food industry is twofold. One, interesterified fats can avoid the negative nutritional publicity of trans fats. Two, it will take years for the dangerous health effects of interesterified fats to be confirmed and reconfirmed (as is often the case in science), and it will take still longer for the FDA to act against them.

Troublesome Enzymes in the Omega-6 and Omega-3 Pathways

The conversion of linoleic acid and alpha-linolenic acid to other members of the omega-6 and omega-3 families, respectively, depends on a handful of enzymes, such as delta-6-desaturase, delta-5-desaturase, elongase, cyclooxygenase 1 and 2, and lipoxygenase. Because the omega-6 and omega-3 fatty acids follow almost parallel biochemical pathways, they depend on many of the same enzymes. (Again, see the illustrations on pages 40 and 41.)

Unfortunately, this dependence on the same enzymes makes the omega-6 and omega-3 pathways competitive, and because the omega-6s are more biologically active, they tend to have an edge and are more likely to promote inflammation. But a number of factors can decrease or increase the activity of these enzymes.

I've already described how trans fats reduce the activity of the D6D enzyme. Alcohol has a similar effect on D6D. Low levels of vitamin B_6, magnesium, and zinc also diminish the effectiveness activity of D6D, in effect slowing or blocking the conversion of linoleic acid to gamma-linoleic acid and of alpha-linolenic acid to stearidonic acid.

Meanwhile, the delta-5-desaturase (D5D) enzyme depends on vitamin C, vitamin B_3, and zinc, and low levels of these nutrients appear to interfere with the production of EPA. In addition, high levels of insulin, found in people with prediabetes, type 2 diabetes, and obesity, increase the activity of D5D—and seem to speed the conversion of dihomo-gamma-linolenic acid to arachidonic acid, leading to greater inflammation. Elevated levels of insulin appear to be common in the two-thirds of Americans who are overweight or obese, 100 million Americans with prediabetes, and 23 million with type 2 diabetes.

Taken as a whole, the research on trans fats shows that they fundamentally alter the body's metabolism of dietary fats and also increase the accumulation of body fat. In addition, they are intertwined with the development of diabetes and heart disease, two conditions that have strong undercurrents of inflammation.

Free Radicals, Antioxidants, and Inflammation

Free radicals, a type of "unbalanced" molecule, have long been known to cause cell damage, leading to degenerative diseases and accelerated aging. They are unbalanced molecules because they have an odd number of subatomic particles called electrons. Typically, electrons come in pairs, and to restore a full pair, a free radical steals an electron from another molecule. That theft damages what had been a healthy cell.

Free radicals are found in virtually all dangerous chemicals, including air pollutants and cigarette smoke, and are generated when your body is exposed to radiation (even from sunlight). They are also created when your body burns food for energy, breaks down harmful chemicals in the liver, or fights infections. Indeed, your body's white blood cells generate large quantities of free radicals to destroy bacteria and virus-infected cells.

Free radicals function as communication molecules that promote or sustain inflammatory reactions. They increase the activity of a substance called "nuclear factor kappa beta," which activates genes involved in inflammation, cancer, and other diseases. Free radicals also boost the activity of interleukin-6, another pro-inflammatory molecule. In addition, free radicals activate several different types of adhesion molecules. Something like a biological glue, these adhesion molecules help white blood cells stick to other cells. Normally, adhesion molecules stick only to germs and damaged cells that are marked for cleanup. But in chronic inflammation, adhesion cells attach to normal cells, such as those in arteries and joints.

Antioxidants Are Anti-Inflammatory

The natural antidotes for free radicals are antioxidants, which include vitamins C and E. Flavonoids, a large family of antioxidants that adds color to vegetables and fruits, are among the most powerful antioxidants. By quenching free radicals, antioxidants also function as anti-inflammatory nutrients. Two extremely effective anti-inflammatory flavonoids are curcumin and Pycnogenol, both of which will be discussed in more detail in chapter 9.

In the next chapter we will see how specific dietary changes have increased our intake of pro-inflammatory omega-6 fatty acids and decreased our consumption of anti-inflammatory omega-3 fatty acids.

CHAPTER 4

Correcting a Diet That's Out of Balance

Although imbalances in fatty acids cause much of a body's overactive inflammatory response, we need to know *why* these imbalances have occurred. The answer is that most people no longer eat many health-promoting and anti-inflammatory foods. Instead, they eat foods that actually stoke the fires of inflammation.

Matt: Treating Multiple Sclerosis with the Original Balanced Diet

In 1995, when Matt was eighteen years old, he suddenly developed severe leg twitches, problems with balance, and an extreme sensitivity to temperature on his left side. One month later, a magnetic resonance imaging scan identified a dozen lesions in his brain and spinal column. The diagnosis was unmistakably multiple sclerosis (MS). Matt envisioned life in a wheelchair—and "almost shut down and gave up," he said.

Matt's dad, Ashton, a scientist, started to read everything about MS he could get hold of—in books, in medical journals, on the Internet. He quickly realized that few researchers and physicians had seriously considered the roles of diet and alternative treatments in controlling MS. Yet such treatments appeared to hold far more promise than drug treatments that were ridden with side effects.

Ashton suggested two therapies to Matt, who was initially skeptical. First came acupuncture. After ten acupuncture treatments, many of Matt's MS symptoms cleared, along with his headaches, night sweats, and allergies. Next came diet. Ashton asked Matt to follow a "Paleolithic," or caveman, diet consisting of simple and unprocessed foods such as fruits, vegetables, fish, skinless chicken breasts, and a little rice, and avoiding all dairy, gluten, legumes, fried foods, and yeast. In addition, Matt began to take a variety of supplements, including vitamins, minerals, omega-3 fatty acids, and GLA.

Since making these changes, Matt has remained completely free of MS symptoms, even while working toward his college degree and then getting a stress-filled job as a television producer. "I stick with the diet religiously," he said. "It was rough for the first six months, but then it became easy. Sure, the foods aren't real exciting, but I would rather use my hand to bring these foods to my mouth than not to be able to use my hand at all. It changed my whole perspective. I don't take as many things for granted."

Nutrients as the Building Blocks of Health

The vital role of nutrition in health is hardly a new idea. Hippocrates, who lived 2,400 years ago and was the father of Western medicine, is remembered by modern physicians for the Hippocratic Oath: first, do no harm (to patients). But Hippocrates' belief that food is our best medicine is now considered little more than a quaint and antiquated concept.

In biology, however, everything revolves around biochemistry. And in biochemistry, all roads (or pathways) ultimately lead back to nutrients. After all, the physical structure of our bodies does not come out of thin air. It is based on a foundation of nutritional biochemicals. For example, the body requires not only calcium to make bone but also vitamins D and K and protein. Similarly, brain development and function require protein, an assortment of vitamins, and ample amounts of healthy fats, including EPA and DHA. Even your genes depend on nutrients, such as the B-complex vitamins for normal functioning, and low levels of these vitamins lead to genetic damage and incorrect messages being transmitted between cells, which can give rise to cancer and other diseases.

Low levels of any nutrient can interfere with a variety of biochemical processes. For example, magnesium plays a role in three hundred biochemical reactions in the body, including some that help control inflammation. Most physicians *assume* the nutritional adequacy of their patients, but it is an assumption that in most cases has no medical basis. It is an assumption because relatively few physicians routinely test their patients' levels of vitamins, minerals, and other nutrients. Without testing, how can one actually be certain? The situation is comparable to a doctor making a casual assumption that a patient's breast lump is not cancerous.

Data from the U.S. Department of Agriculture and other reputable organizations and universities have found nutritional deficiencies to be common in the United States. Three-fourths of Americans consume suboptimal amounts of folic acid, a B vitamin needed for normal gene function and to prevent heart disease and cancer. Indeed, studies published in 2009 found that three of every four Americans do not have adequate levels of vitamin D, and these widespread "insufficiencies" and outright deficiences significantly increase the risk of osteoporosis, cancer, heart disease, muscle wasting, and depression. Although many people consume excess sugars and sugarlike carbohydrates, most do not obtain the minimal requirements for vitamins and minerals.

The result is that people essentially limp through life, biochemically and nutritionally, not feeling as well as they could if their nutritional intake was optimal. Chronic inflammation is one of the signs that things are amiss—and that there is room for improvement in both nutrition and health.

Rediscovering Our Original Diet

There is a perennial controversy about the ideal diet for people. In fact, there is no shortage of diets or eating recommendations—high protein, low carb, low fat, high carb, and gluten free, to name just a few. Advocates of particular diets often express a near-religious insistence on the righteousness of their diet versus others. So how does one make sense of all of the different diet and eating plans?

I believe our biological past offers important clues for a baseline (that is, a starting point) anti-inflammatory diet, which we can tweak and adapt to our modern lifestyles and individual needs. The idea behind our distant ancestral diet (also known as our evolutionary, Paleolithic, or Stone Age diet) is fairly straightforward. Over millions of years, human beings developed in a biological milieu that provided certain nutrients, which became essential for life and health. This nutritional environment helped shape our genes and biology. So when we look to the past, it's important to consider both what our ancestors ate and what they did not eat.

It turns out that our genes are virtually identical to those of people who lived roughly 10,000 to 40,000 years ago. Indeed, our genes have changed relatively little—only about 0.5 percent—during the 2 million previous years. We are, biologically, cavemen and cavewomen, but most of us now eat food products that did not exist until very recently. These dietary changes make us more prone to developing inflammatory disorders.

Evolutionary vs. Modern Diets

Until relatively recently, understanding the Paleolithic diet was largely the province of anthropologists and archaeologists who worked in relative obscurity at museums and universities. In 1985, S. Boyd Eaton, M.D., of Emory University, Atlanta, and his anthropologist colleagues published a watershed article in the *New England Journal of Medicine* that gave new credibility to ancient nutrition.

Since that time, Eaton and his colleagues, as well as Loren Cordain, Ph.D., of Colorado State University, the author of *The Paleo Diet*, have greatly expanded our understanding of the Paleolithic diet and how it differs from our modern diets. These scientists have based their ideas on a vast body of archaeological evidence, including bones, coprolites, and food remains at prehistoric sites, as well as detailed ethnographic records of 229 "hunter-gatherer" cultures that existed through the nineteenth or twentieth centuries.

Paleolithic people lived before the advent of agriculture, the intentional growing of crops. For sustenance, they hunted large and small game animals, fished in rivers or oceans, and foraged a variety of plant foods, including leaves, roots, fruits, seeds, and nuts. As you might imagine, living without modern conveniences was hard and life expectancies were short, with injuries and infections being the leading causes of death. Yet the archaeological record indicates that these primitive people were generally healthier than people are today, and they rarely experienced our modern diseases, such as arthritis, heart disease, and cancer.

It is important to note that the "typical" Paleolithic diet is a composite of many different diets, just as the average American (Western) diet is also a composite. In addition, although Paleolithic food choices varied by geography and season, they were often consistent in macronutrient (protein, carbohydrate, fat) and micronutrient (vitamin and mineral) levels, as well as in the foods *not* eaten. Despite the differences in geography, Paleolithic peoples were sophisticated hunters and gatherers, and they consumed an extraordinarily diverse selection of meats, fish (if they lived near oceans or lakes), and vegetables.

Mary Jo: Back from the Brink

Mary Jo, who lives near Oklahoma City, Oklahoma, suddenly became "deathly ill," and her husband rushed her to the emergency room. The doctors knew something was seriously wrong—her liver enzymes were abnormally high—but they had difficulty pinpointing the cause. Exploratory surgery found that Mary Jo's liver was as "hard as a rock," as she described it.

Mary Jo had developed cirrhosis caused by a chronic hepatitis C infection that she didn't even know she had. She had lived the "clean life" and suspected that she had contracted hepatitis C from a contaminated blood transfusion forty years earlier. The doctors said she had two months to live, maybe up to a year if she started interferon therapy. "But I talked with other patients, and the side effects scared me," she said.

As Mary Jo scrambled to read everything she could on the subject, she learned about Burt Berkson, M.D., Ph.D., a nutritionally oriented physician and an expert in liver diseases. By the time she got to Berkson's clinic in Las Cruces, New Mexico, she couldn't walk without another person holding her up. Her voice was so weak, she couldn't speak above a whisper. (See the section on "Hepatitis" in chapter 12.)

Berkson knew from experience exactly what to do. He put Mary Jo on a "natural and conservative" high-potency liver-boosting, anti-inflammatory regimen—alpha-lipoic acid, silymarin (*Silybum marianum*), and selenium. He also coached Mary Jo on how to improve her eating habits, with an emphasis on fresh and whole foods.

Two weeks later, Mary Jo was ready to take on the world. As soon as she returned home, she began to clean the house, do laundry, and tackle other chores, and a few months later she power-washed and painted her house. "I got my energy back," she said in a clear, strong voice. "And today I do anything I want to do."

We Need Protein

Protein forms the foundation of our physical structure—that is, our muscles, organs, glands, and, to a great extent, our bones and teeth. The components of protein are also needed by the body to synthesize DNA, hormones, neurochemicals, and other biochemicals, including those involved in pro- and anti-inflammatory reactions.

There is no evidence of an entirely vegetarian or even mostly vegetarian hunter-gatherer society. Paleolithic and hunter-gatherer societies preferred animal foods, including fish, over plant foods, according to the latest research by Cordain. Nearly three-fourths (73 percent) of hunter-gatherer societies worldwide obtained more than half of their food from animals. In contrast, only about one-eighth (14 percent) of societies obtained more than half of their food from plants. Indeed, many anthropologists believe that the development of agriculture became a necessity because human populations had overhunted large game.

The typical Paleolithic intake of protein ranged from 19 to 35 percent of people's calories and sometimes as much as 50 percent of their calories. In general, the amount of animal foods increased and plant foods decreased in the diets of people living farther from the equator. (Long-term intake of a diet containing more than 50 percent protein can be toxic, and Cordain believes that hunter-gatherers balanced a very high protein intake by increasing their consumption of animal fat.) In contrast, the typical American adult obtains about 15 percent of his or her calories from protein, substantially less than Paleolithic peoples and hunter-gatherer societies.

We Need Fats

Like protein, fats have multiple roles. They help form the walls of cells and regulate what enters and exits those cells, and they are also an integral part of almost all body tissues and many biochemicals. As you have already read, fats form the building blocks of the body's pro- and anti-inflammatory compounds.

Paleolithic peoples and hunter-gatherer societies consumed 28 to 58 percent of their calories in the form of fat, a quantity that is for the most part higher than the average intake of 34 percent today. Despite the large amount of fat, the specific types of fat were very different in Paleolithic times—and far more balanced in terms of inflammation-promoting or inflammation-suppressing fats. The ratio of omega-6 (inflammation-promoting) to omega-3 (inflammation-suppressing) fatty acids in the diet ranged from about 1:1 to 2:1.

Meat from wild game, the mainstay of most Paleolithic peoples and hunter-gatherer societies, is considerably leaner than is meat from modern domesticated cattle. For example, grass-fed cattle (whose diet would be similar to that of wild game) have six to eight times less fat than do grain-fed cattle. Furthermore, beef from grass-fed cattle has two to six times more omega-3 fatty acids, compared with meat from grain-fed cattle. A similar pattern occurs in other types of livestock. Grass-fed bison have seven times more omega-3 fatty acids than do grain-fed bison. The grasses and leaves eaten by animals contain substantial amounts of omega-3 fatty acids, which are eventually deposited in the animals' muscles and fat. When people eat such meats, as they did in the past, they consume these anti-inflammatory omega-3 fatty acids.

Today's domesticated livestock are typically fed cereal grains (such as corn) for several months before slaughter, increasing their overall fat, saturated fat, and pro-inflammatory arachidonic acid. Such meat contains low levels of omega-3 fatty acids, leading to a high ratio of omega-6 to omega-3 fatty acids. For example, about 3 percent of the fat in wild game consists of omega-3 fatty acids, but only 0.4 percent (less than one-seventh the amount) of the fat in grain-fed beef does. So when people consume meat from grain-fed domesticated animals, the lopsided omega-6 to omega-3 ratio further contributes to their pro-inflammatory profile.

Perhaps surprisingly, cholesterol consumption has not changed significantly since Paleolithic times. Elevated cholesterol levels per se are not necessarily problematic, but they can become pro-inflammatory when combined with a low intake of antioxidants, such as in a diet with few vegetables and fruits.

Based on an analysis of 829 plants, wild plant foods contain an average of 24 percent fat, a surprisingly large amount. Such plants, as well as modern leafy green vegetables (kale, spinach, dark green lettuces, greens), contain substantial amounts of alpha-linolenic acid, the building block of the omega-3 fatty acids. In ancient times, this mix of natural, uncultivated plant foods and wild game meat led to a balanced intake of omega-6 and omega-3 fatty acids, which tempered inflammatory responses.

Especially significant, Paleolithic peoples and later hunter-gatherer societies did not consume *any* oils or fats unless they were part of meat or vegetables. Our ancestors *never* consumed pressed or refined oils. This contrasts sharply with today, with corn, soy, and safflower oil—all rich in pro-inflammatory omega-6 fatty acids—being ubiquitous in kitchens and packaged foods. These oils, often manipulated to mimic saturated fats and to form trans-fatty acids, are used to lubricate fry pans and to deep-fry potatoes, chicken, and fish and are added to the vast majority of processed (packaged) foods, such as salad dressings, microwave meals, meat extenders, baked goods, and chocolate bars.

Switching from a diet that is high in saturated fat to one high in omega-6 fatty acids—the very change that public health authorities have recommended to Americans during the last thirty years—actually decreases the body's production of anti-inflammatory omega-3 compounds (specifically, EPA and DHA) by 40 to 50 percent. In addition, many foods, such as fried potatoes and fried chicken, are cooked in oxidized vegetable oils, increasing their content of free radicals and adding to the pro-inflammatory burden.

We Need Carbohydrates and Fiber

Carbohydrates, made up of starches and sugars, provide most of the body's energy—that is, they are burned for fuel or stored as fat. In Paleolithic times and in hunter-gatherer societies, carbohydrates came almost entirely from uncultivated high-fiber, low-starch vegetables (leaves, shoots, buds, roots), fruit, seeds, and nuts. The carbohydrates in uncultivated and unprocessed vegetables are complex, meaning that they are digested slowly, in contrast to simple sugars and refined starches (such as those in breads and pastas), which are absorbed rapidly. Complex carbohydrates are part of the plant's matrix, which includes substantial amounts of protein, vitamins, minerals, and fiber. In other words, Paleolithic peoples and hunter-gatherer societies ate relatively low-carbohydrate diets, and the carbohydrates were not readily absorbed.

Today, only a minority of people regularly consume substantive amounts of vegetables and fruit daily. Instead, the vast majority of dietary carbohydrates and calories come from highly refined grains (chiefly wheat but also corn and rye), sugars (sucrose and high-fructose corn syrup, particularly in soft drinks and other beverages), and fried potatoes (which contain trans-fatty acids and oxidized omega-6 fatty acids).

One excellent marker of vegetable intake is dietary fiber content. In Paleolithic times, people ate an average of 100 grams of fiber daily from vegetables and fruit. Today, the typical Westerner eats only 20 grams daily, mostly from grains. Although whole grains, such as whole-wheat bread, provide some vitamins, minerals, and fiber, they still fall far short of vegetables in the amount of vitamins, minerals, and fiber they contain. And as grain consumption has increased over the years, vegetable and fruit consumption has decreased.

The effect of refined grains and sugars on inflammation is significant, though not as obvious as with oils and fats. Consumption of refined grains and sugars typically raises blood sugar levels and, over the long term, increases the risk of diabetes. Researchers have found that very modest chronic rises in blood sugar, even when in the normal range, significantly increase the risk of developing diabetes or heart disease within just a few years. Both diseases have inflammatory undercurrents, and elevations in blood sugar generate free radicals, which can stimulate inflammation.

We Need Vitamins, Minerals, and Phytonutrients

Over the course of a typical year, Paleolithic peoples and hunter-gatherer societies consumed more than a hundred types of plants. These were very different foods from what most people consume today. Ancient uncultivated vegetables were more akin to nutrient-packed kale than to iceberg lettuce, and uncultivated fruit looked more like crabapples and rose hips than supersweet pears and bananas.

Only 9 to 32 percent of North Americans consume the five daily servings of vegetables and fruit recommended by the federal government, meaning that 68 to 91 percent of Americans do not eat a particularly rich dietary source of vitamins and other micronutrients. Of those people who do eat vegetables and fruit, most choose from a limited selection, such as potatoes, which are often fried; corn; peas; carrots; and iceberg lettuce. As a consequence, most people today fall far short of the greater quantity and diversity of vitamins, minerals, and phytonutrients consumed by Paleolithic peoples and hunter-gatherers.

Based on the calculations by Eaton and Cordain, Paleolithic humans consumed an average of two to ten times more vitamins and minerals than people do today. These levels range from three to six times the federal government's Recommended Dietary Allowance (or Daily Value) for vitamins and minerals. For example, a Paleolithic person likely ingested about 600 mg of vitamin C daily, compared with an RDA of 60 mg and a typical North American daily intake of 45 mg or less daily.

In addition, vegetables and fruit contain large amounts of vitamin-like antioxidant nutrients, particularly flavonoids and carotenoids. A diet containing a diverse selection of vegetables and fruit would likely provide hundreds of flavonoids and dozens of carotenoids. Researchers estimate that people nowadays consume between 23 and 170 mg of flavonoids daily, but that they may have consumed five to twenty-four times more (115 to 4,080 mg daily) in the past. Such a huge dietary intake of antioxidants—now missing from most people's diets—would certainly moderate inflammatory reactions.

—∿—

Past and Present Intake of Vitamins and Minerals

VITAMINS	PALEOLITHIC* (MG/DAY)	CURRENT U.S.† (MG/DAY)	RATIO
Vitamin C	604	93	6.5
Vitamin E	32.8	8.5	3.9
Vitamin B_2	6.49	1.71	3.8
Vitamin B_1	3.91	1.42	2.8
Vitamin A	17.2	7.8	2.2
Folic acid	0.36	0.18	2

MINERALS	PALEOLITHIC* (MG/DAY)	CURRENT U.S.† (MG/DAY)	RATIO
Copper	12.2	1.2	10.2
Iron	87.4	10.5	8.3
Manganese	13.3	3	4.4
Potassium	10,500	2,500	4.2
Magnesium	1,223	320	3.8
Zinc	43.4	12.5	3.5
Phosphorus	3,223	1,510	2.1
Calcium	1,622	920	1.8
Sodium	768	4,000	0.2

* Based on 3,000 calories daily, 35 percent animal and 65 percent plant subsistence.
† Average of U.S. men and women; Food and Nutrition Board, 1989.

—∿—

The Turning Points in Our Diet

Americans, and increasingly Canadians and Europeans, certainly do enjoy full stomachs. The latest statistics show that three of every four Americans are overweight and half of those are obese—at least thirty pounds over their ideal weight. Being overweight is not a sign of good nutrition; rather, it is a sign of excessive calorie and carbohydrate intake, usually at the expense of more nutrient-dense and wholesome foods.

There are many ways to look at the history of dietary changes and to analyze how these changes affect people's health. Because this book is about inflammation, the emphasis in our brief examination of food history will be on how the diet has shifted from relatively balanced to clearly pro-inflammatory. Three major periods of dietary change have occurred: the agricultural revolution, the industrial revolution, and the convenience/fast-food revolution. All of these changes have been characterized by two basic trends: (1) through a variety of processing and refining methods, the modern diet less and less resembles our evolutionary diet, and (2) the majority of foods sold in supermarkets less and less resemble their original appearance in nature.

The Agricultural Diet

The first major changes to the diet—that is, a departure from lean meat, fish, and vegetables, nuts, seeds, and fruits—occurred approximately 10,000 years ago with the development of agriculture, the domestication of livestock, and the use of milk and other dairy products. Agriculture stabilized the movement of hunter-gatherer societies, which eventually led to the growth of cities and the development of complex cultures. But the use of grains and dairy products also led to health problems that were not immediately evident.

The cultivation and consumption of grains introduced the protein gluten to the diet of humans. Gluten is an umbrella term for forty related proteins in a handful of grains, specifically wheat, rye, and barley. You might think that a new vegetarian source of protein would be good, but gluten has been a mixed blessing.

Approximately one in every hundred people is allergic to gluten, causing celiac disease. In these people, eating gluten triggers an immune (inflammatory) response, which primarily attacks the gastrointestinal tract and interferes with vitamin and mineral absorption. Archaeologists have noted that the health of humans, based largely on the analysis of ancient bones, took a turn for the worse after gluten-containing grains entered the diet. Osteoporosis, arthritis, and even birth defects became more common after people began eating grains.

The health effects of gluten proteins in grains may even be problematic for many people who do not have celiac disease. Half of Westerners may be sensitive to gluten without exhibiting any of the traditional symptoms of celiac disease. Instead, gluten sensitivity may appear as immunological reactions affecting the nervous system, balance, and behavior, as well as a person's overall sense of well-being. Meanwhile, a second family of grain (and legume) proteins, called lectins, may also damage the gut and interfere with nutrient absorption. In addition, lectins might play a role in rheumatoid arthritis and other inflammatory autoimmune diseases. The bottom line is that most grains are neither the much-heralded staff of life nor the breakfast of champions.

Ten millennia ago—too short a time for genetic evolution—people also began to domesticate livestock for meat and, in the case of cows and goats, for milk and other dairy products. As long as livestock were exclusively grass-fed, their meat and milk yielded a balance of pro- and anti-inflammatory fatty acids. This changed when animals were fed corn, which, as previously noted, increases the animals' overall fat and saturated fat and reduces anti-inflammatory omega-3 fatty acids.

Many people have questioned the health benefits of cow's milk, but a couple of points are especially relevant in the context of our evolutionary diet. One is that no species, other than humans over the last 10,000 years, has ever consumed milk beyond infancy. Another is that no species other than humans has ever consumed the milk of another mammal. Like grains, cow's milk appears to be a mismatch for our genetic heritage.

—⁂—

Some Differences between Paleolithic and Modern Diets

FOOD GROUP	PALEOLITHIC	MODERN
Protein	Very lean	Fatty
Carbohydrates	From vegetables	From grains and refined sugars
Fats	Balanced intake	Pro-inflammatory
FOOD TYPES		
Animal/fish foods*	65 percent of diet	15 percent of diet
Vegetables/fruit	About 100 different plants	Very narrow selection
Fiber	100 grams daily	20 grams daily
Vitamins/minerals	Substantially more	Substantially less
Grains	None	Substantial intake
Dairy	None	Substantial intake
Pressed oils	None	Substantial intake
Trans fats	Negligible	Substantial intake
Alcohol	None	3 percent of calories

* Animal and fish foods were not exclusively protein. These foods also supplied fat and bone.

—⁂—

The Industrial Diet

Many dietary changes occurred over the next ten millennia, including a greater cultivation of vegetables and fruit, which increased the sugar content and reduced the bitterness of produce. But perhaps the most significant changes relate to the refining of wheat, which has become a staple food. The use of new technologies to refine grains as well as sugars foreshadowed many other changes.

In the nineteenth century, metal rollers replaced stone grinding wheels (grindstones), enabling millers to achieve a more mechanized and efficient means of processing grains into flour. Grains could be processed faster, yielding much finer flour, without bits of stone being eroded from grinding wheels and ending up in the flour. In addition, the new technologies enabled easier separation of the grain's germ and bran from the endosperm, which was mostly carbohydrate. The nutrient-lacking endosperm was used for baking bread and other products, whereas the germ and the bran were often fed to livestock. In addition, the endosperm-based flour used in baking was bleached chemically to make it white, increasing its consumer appeal.

The industrialization of the grain-refining process yielded "white bread" for the masses instead of only for a limited number of wealthy people. Nutritionally, the difference between whole-grain and white bread was disastrous. During the 1930s, increasing consumption of white bread contributed to deficiencies of several B vitamins in North America and Europe. The situation led to government-mandated "enrichment" of flours to replace a handful of the many nutrients removed during grain refining.

The Convenience/Fast-Food Diet

After the end of World War II, technologists helped guide unprecedented prosperity in the United States. The first Swanson brand TV dinner, a frozen meal on a metal tray, was introduced in 1953, heralding the start of the convenience/fast-food revolution. It was a commercial success. Several years later, in southern California, automobiles and food intersected, giving rise to McDonald's and the fast-food industry. The trade-off for fast, convenient food was lower nutritional value and fewer anti-inflammatory nutrients.

Meanwhile, more women entered the workforce and had less time than before to prepare large home-cooked meals (with most men not helping in the kitchen). The need to reduce time in the kitchen fueled the popularity of the microwave oven in the 1970s. TV dinners that baked in the oven for forty minutes were replaced by microwave meals that were ready in five minutes. For the first time in history, large numbers of people did not have to wait very long, or expend much effort, before sitting down and eating. This was a major change from when people spent their entire days hunting and gathering food and burning off calories in the process.

The economic climate of the 1990s reinforced the demand for convenience and fast—and faster—food. The pace of business quickened with the pressures of international competition, overnight deliveries, and e-mail. People who had once comfortably ended their workday at 5:00 P.M. are now connected to their offices 24/7 via e-mail, cell phones, and texting. More and more, fast and convenience foods have become the way to sandwich meals into hectic schedules.

For the most part, these meals are made with ingredients that are high in refined carbohydrates and pro-inflammatory omega-6 and trans-fatty acids and very low in vitamins, minerals, fiber, omega-3s, and protein. A recent study published in the *Journal of the American Dietetic Association* found that two-thirds of the carbohydrates consumed by U.S. adults come from bread, soft drinks, cakes and cookies, refined cereal, pasta, cooked grains, and ice cream. These refined carbohydrates raise blood sugar levels, creating a prediabetic or diabeticlike blood profile, which generates pro-inflammatory free radicals. Recent research by Simin Liu, M.D., Ph.D., of Harvard Medical School, has consistently found that diets high in refined carbohydrates and high-glycemic foods (which rapidly raise blood sugar levels) increase inflammation. In one of Liu's studies, women eating large amounts of potatoes, breakfast cereals, white bread, muffins, and white rice had elevated C-reactive protein levels, indicating high levels of inflammation. Overweight women who ate a lot of these foods had the highest and most dangerous CRP levels. All of these carbohydrates (and the fats they are often combined with) displace far healthier foods, such as anti-inflammatory vegetables, fruit, and fish.

Another inflammation-promoting substance forms when foods are cooked at high temperatures. Advanced glycation end products (AGEs) are created when sugars bind in a particular way to proteins. As the acronym suggests, AGEs accelerate the aging process. AGEs also increase levels of C-reactive protein, a powerful promoter of inflammation. In a study with diabetic patients, those who consumed foods cooked at high temperatures had a 65 percent increase in AGEs after just two weeks. Yet, people eating the same foods cooked at low temperatures had a 30 percent decrease in AGEs. The AGE-lowering foods were cooked by boiling or steaming—or were quickly sautéed with a small amount of oil. Baking foods for hours, such as how the typical Thanksgiving turkey is prepared, generates large amounts of AGEs. In addition, coffee, cola drinks, chocolate drinks, and fried foods are very high in AGEs.

What is the bottom line with all of these refined, processed foods? First, they displace many important nutrients, such as anti-inflammatory vitamins, minerals, protein, and omega-3 fatty acids. Second, many grains interfere with normal nutrient absorption. Third, highly refined sugars and carbohydrates draw nutrients such as vitamins and minerals from the body's reserves to aid the metabolic processes that normally burn these foods for energy. Fourth, the sheer quantity of calories and carbohydrates in refined sugars and carbohydrates promotes obesity, and fat cells generate large amounts of interleukin-6 and C-reactive protein, two of the most powerful pro-inflammatory compounds made by the body.

The end result is a diet that's high in pro-inflammatory fats, devoid of anti-inflammatory fats, and nearly empty of anti-inflammatory anti-oxidants.

And anti-inflammatory drugs don't really help, as we'll see in the next chapter.

CHAPTER 5

What's Wrong with Anti-Inflammatory Drugs

Melinda: When the Cure Is Worse Than the Disease

You might think that "iatrogenic disease" is some sort of rare condition. But the term actually refers to any illness caused by a physician or a treatment. And it's surprisingly common. In a typical year, more than 100,000 hospitalized patients die from medications they had been prescribed, and more than 2 million others suffer severe side effects. Incredibly, no one knows the number of serious adverse reactions and deaths that occur from over-the-counter medications and prescription drugs.

When Melinda was in her midthirties, she sought more aggressive medical treatment of her allergies and asthma, as well as of her increasingly stiff joints. Up to this point, she had used either over-the-counter or prescription antihistamines for her allergies, nasal corticosteroid hormones for her asthma, and ibuprofen (an NSAID, or nonsteroidal anti-inflammatory drug) for her rheumatoid arthritis.

Melinda's physician put her on prednisone, a hormone treatment for allergies and arthritis and a potent prescription-strength NSAID. Side effects from the prednisone included a seventy-pound weight gain, weakened bones, and increased susceptibility to colds and flus, which left Melinda feeling tired much of the time. The NSAID caused a painful gastric ulcer, which was treated by a drug to reduce stomach acid.

The medications and Melinda's weight gain substantially increased her risk of developing heart disease and, particularly, heart failure (a catastrophic weakening of the heart muscle). Melinda's physician tried to head off the damage, but he relied solely on pharmaceutical treatments and never discussed nutrition or an anti-inflammatory diet with her. Two years later, after a battery of laboratory tests, he noted that her C-reactive protein levels were elevated, a sign of serious inflammation, so he prescribed a cholesterol-lowering "statin" drug to reduce her risk of developing heart disease.

The statin drug lowered Melinda's cholesterol, but it also decreased her body's production of coenzyme Q_{10}, a vitaminlike substance needed for normal heart function. Both the statin and the NSAID increased her risk of suffering heart failure. As Melinda's heart function declined, her physician prescribed one more drug to stimulate the heart.

Sadly, her downward spiral could not be stopped. Melinda died of heart failure at age thirty-nine, even though her symptoms could have been reversed by diet and safe nutritional supplements.

With dozens of over-the-counter and prescription anti-inflammatory drugs on the market, you might think that the cure for your aches and pains is as near as the corner pharmacy. Many of these drugs, such as aspirin and ibuprofen, provide relief to millions of people around the world. But these and other drugs have a dark side that, perhaps in the majority of cases, outweighs their benefits. In this chapter we will look at the hazards of several classes of anti-inflammatory drugs.

Anti-Inflammatory Drugs and Their Hazards

Pharmaceutical drugs, used appropriately and for short periods of time, can quickly relieve pain and inflammation. Yet they are anything but magic bullets. The longer such drugs are used, and this is the case with chronic inflammatory diseases, the greater the risk of serious side effects occurring.

Drug companies market more than 30 different types of NSAIDs, the most widely used class of drugs. Many other drugs are also used to treat inflammation, and 250 are sold for the treatment of arthritis alone. Each year, pharmacists in the United States fill more than 70 million prescriptions for NSAIDs, and consumers buy about 30 billion over-the-counter NSAID products. According to an article in the *New England Journal of Medicine*, NSAID complications lead to 7,500 bleeding ulcers, 103,000 hospitalizations, and 16,500 deaths annually, costing more than $2 billion in medical expenses.

Three classes of medications are used to treat inflammatory diseases, and a fourth is rapidly emerging. These medications are corticosteroids, conventional over-the-counter and prescription NSAIDs, the first generation of selective Cox-2-inhibiting NSAIDs, and the relatively new use of "statin" drugs to reduce C-reactive protein levels.

Corticosteroids

Introduced in the 1950s, cortisonelike drugs called corticosteroids or glucocorticoids remain extraordinarily popular. These drugs are synthetic mimics of stress-response hormones produced in the adrenal glands. Physicians can choose among dozens of corticosteroids to treat inflammation, but perhaps the best-known corticosteroid is prednisone, which is sold under a variety of brand names.

Corticosteroids are frequently the first treatment that physicians prescribe to patients diagnosed with autoimmune diseases such as rheumatoid arthritis, asthma, lupus erythematosus, or multiple sclerosis. They rapidly and dramatically dampen the body's overactive immune response and sometimes are necessary as a *brief* intervention. That's the good news. The bad news about prednisone and other corticosteroids reads like a chamber of medical horrors. Over several weeks or months, oral or injected corticosteroids affect almost every organ and lead to serious side effects while the drugs are being taken, as well as cause permanent damage.

Among the most common side effects is a rounded "moon face," which is considered characteristic of prednisone use. An increase in abdominal obesity is also common. Because prednisone and other corticosteroids dampen the immune response, they increase susceptibility to infection, often masking symptoms of active infections, and they interfere with the normal healing of wounds. As a consequence, when people take corticosteroids for many weeks or months, their cuts, scrapes, and more serious injuries are slow to heal.

Corticosteroids also interfere with the metabolism of key nutrients, including folic acid, vitamins B_6 and B_{12}, potassium, and zinc. Because these drugs also reduce vitamin D and calcium levels, they prevent normal bone development in young people. In adults, long-term use of corticosteroids leads to decreased bone density and osteoporosis. Some corticosteroids can be injected directly into the joints of people with arthritis, but repeated injections accelerate joint damage.

Other common side effects of corticosteroids include a thinning of the skin and bruising, high blood pressure, elevated blood sugar levels (which increase the risk of developing diabetes and coronary artery disease), cataracts and glaucoma, male infertility, menstrual irregularities, and loss of muscle mass.

Conventional NSAIDs

Aspirin, ibuprofen (Advil, Motrin, and generic brands), and naproxen sodium (Aleve and others) are the most popular over-the-counter nonsteroidal anti-inflammatory drugs, and many higher-potency NSAIDs are available by prescription. The term *NSAID* means that these drugs are anti-inflammatory but are not based on steroid hormones. NSAIDs are very effective in relieving headaches, controlling inflammation, easing pain, and reducing fevers. But like other anti-inflammatory drugs, they pose considerable dangers, particularly when used regularly.

Aspirin, which has been widely used since about 1900, is the oldest pharmaceutical NSAID. Before aspirin was synthesized, people often used willow bark, which contains a compound very similar to synthetic aspirin. For many years, researchers believed that NSAIDs worked by inhibiting the activity of cyclooxygenase, an enzyme that is essential for the conversion of fatty acids to pro- and anti-inflammatory compounds. In the early 1990s, researchers discovered a second form of cyclooxygenase, so the two compounds are now referred to as Cox-1 and Cox-2. The prevailing view in medicine has been that Cox-1, whose levels are generally steady, performs normal cell functions. In contrast, doctors have believed that Cox-2 levels rise as part of the body's inflammatory response.

In the course of research, scientists quickly realized that most NSAIDs interfere with both Cox-1 and Cox-2, causing a variety of side effects in many people. The most common side effect of NSAIDs is an upset stomach, which affects at least 10 to 20 percent of people taking these drugs, but according to some studies may affect up to 50 percent of users. In 10 to 25 percent of people regularly taking NSAIDs, the stomach wall erodes, leading to gastritis (inflammation of the stomach wall) and the formation of gastric ulcers. Ironically, as physicians have successfully treated *Helicobacter pylori* infections, a major cause of stomach ulcers, NSAIDs have become the leading cause of ulcers. The reason is NSAIDs' suppression of Cox-1, which is essential for maintaining the integrity of stomach and duodenal (the upper part of the intestine, just below the stomach) walls. Cox-1 is also important in the body's anti-inflammatory processes.

Aspirin is also a potent anticoagulant, largely because it interferes with chemicals involved in blood clotting. Many physicians recommend a very small amount of aspirin daily to reduce the long-term risk of developing coronary artery disease. But aspirin's blood-thinning effect also increases the tendency toward bleeding (such as in nosebleeds) and bleeding time, making wounds slower to close and heal.

Two lines of research indicate that NSAIDs can be even more dangerous. A recent study published in *Archives of Internal Medicine* found that the regular use of NSAIDs (except for aspirin) doubles a person's risk of being hospitalized for heart failure. Physicians John Page, M.B.B.S., and David Henry, M.B.ChB., of the University of Newcastle, Australia, found that NSAID use among seniors with a history of heart disease increased the risk of hospitalization for heart failure by ten times. Seniors are the biggest users of NSAIDs, chiefly for rheumatoid arthritis, osteoarthritis, and other aches and pains. Page and Henry calculated that NSAID use might account for almost one-fifth of all hospital admissions for heart failure, one of the most serious of all heart diseases.

The other mind-boggling feature of regular NSAID use is that some of these drugs, particularly aspirin and ibuprofen, actually *accelerate* the breakdown of cartilage in joints. This is especially ironic among people who take NSAIDs to relieve the pain of osteoarthritis, a disease characterized by the destruction of cartilage padding in the joints. Despite the fact that this breakdown of joint cartilage is very well documented, few patients are ever told of it. Although acetaminophen is not an NSAID, it appears to have a similar effect on promoting osteoarthritis.

Cox-2 Inhibitors

With the discovery of two forms of cyclooxygenase enzymes, and the mistaken belief that only the Cox-2 enzyme was involved in inflammation, several pharmaceutical companies began massive research projects to develop a new generation of Cox-2 inhibitors. In theory, these drugs would stop inflammation by suppressing Cox-2 activity but would avoid the gastrointestinal side effects associated with the inhibition of Cox-1.

Celebrex and Vioxx were the first "selective" Cox-2 inhibitors. But the new generation of Cox-2 inhibitors (often referred to as "coxibs") was only 20 percent selective for Cox-2. In other words, they were 80 percent nonselective, just like traditional NSAIDs. Coxibs were no more effective therapeutically and no safer than earlier NSAIDs.

One early study, testing Vioxx against naproxen, found that the Cox-2 inhibitor increased the incidence of heart attack by four times, compared with the older NSAID. A later analysis of four studies of Cox-2 inhibitors confirmed that this new class of drugs increases the risk of suffering heart attack and stroke, according to an article in the *Journal of the American Medical Association*.

It was a sign of things to come. Merck, the giant drug company that developed Vioxx, kept defending the drug. But new studies showed that Vioxx doubled the risk of heart attacks and stroke, and it became clear that Merck had released only positive (while hiding the negative) findings from its studies to influence the prescribing habits of physicians. In September 2004, as the Food and Drug Administration was about to ban Vioxx, Merck withdrew the drug from the market. More than 80 million people had been given prescriptions for Vioxx, and the U.S. Food and Drug Administration has estimated that 88,000 to 139,000 people suffered heart attacks from the drug, about 30 to 40 percent of which were fatal. By all indications, Celebrex (which is still sold on prescription) also seems to increase the risk of cardiovascular disease, although not to the same degree as Vioxx. Meanwhile, in 2005, the drug Bextra (valdecoxib) was withdrawn from the market as well, because of dangerous side effects.

The fiasco surrounding Vioxx shows the dangers of both pharmaceutical thinking and a limited understanding of human biochemistry. Drug companies develop drugs they can patent, whereas natural products such as omega-3 fish oils and gamma-linolenic acid cannot be easily patented. Using Vioxx amounted to throwing a wrench into the body's inflammatory machinery, whereas taking the omega-3s and gamma-linolenic acid would have been a more straightforward and biochemically sound, but less profitable, way to control inflammation.

Researchers have discovered that Cox-2 has diverse fundamental roles in human biology, aside from its role in inflammation. Like Cox-1, Cox-2 is necessary in maintaining the integrity of the stomach wall, as well as normal kidney and blood platelet function. In addition, Cox-2 appears to be active in brain development, activity, and memory. It is also involved in ovulation and the implantation of the egg into the womb. So it should come as no surprise that using drugs to suppress Cox-2 leads to undesirable side effects. Furthermore, because the so-called "selective Cox-2 inhibitors" aren't much different from traditional NSAIDs, they affect the activity of Cox-1, which is needed to make anti-inflammatory prostaglandin E_1 and E_3.

CRP-Lowering Agents

Most recently, pharmaceutical companies have repositioned their cholesterol-lowering statin drugs as ways to also lower levels of C-reactive protein. These drugs include Lipitor (atorvastatin), Mevacor (lovastatin), Pravachol (pravastatin), Zocor (simvastatin), Crestor (rosuvastatin), and Vytorin (combining simvastatin with ezetimibe). Another statin, Baycol (cerivastatin), was taken off the market because of dangerous side effects. These drugs make big money for their makers. Lipitor alone now earns the drug company Pfizer more than $13 billion annually.

Although many studies have found that vitamin E and other nutrients significantly reduce CRP levels, several major pharmaceutical trials have begun to position "statin" drugs as the therapy of choice for lowering CRP levels.

In 2008, a study published in the *New England Journal of Medicine* was the most aggressive attempt (to date) at positioning a statin drug, specifically Crestor, as a treatment for chronic low-grade inflammation. The study, called JUPITER, tracked almost 18,000 subjects with normal cholesterol levels but high levels of C-reactive protein. The report garnered newspaper headlines because Crestor apparently reduced the risk of suffering heart attack and stroke by half.

But these findings were in many ways a distortion of the research. It is true that Crestor reduced inflammation and cut the "relative risk" of heart attack or stroke by half. But when looked at in terms of "absolute risk," or real-world risk, only 1 person of every 120 benefited from the drug. Worse, far more people—25 percent in real-world terms—taking Crestor developed type 2 diabetes, compared with people taking placebos.

Despite their popularity and a common perception of safety, statins pose other serious risks. They reduce the body's production of cholesterol by inhibiting an enzyme known as HMG-CoA-reductase. This enzyme is active in a series of biochemical reactions that eventually leads to the production of cholesterol (which, by the way, is the core molecule in all of the body's steroid hormones, including estrogen, testosterone, and corticosteroids). The problem is that statins also turn off the body's production of all of the other compounds that depend on HMG-CoA-reductase.

One of these downstream compounds is coenzyme Q_{10} (CoQ_{10}). CoQ_{10} is a vitaminlike substance that plays a pivotal role in how the body's cells produce energy. CoQ_{10} is so crucial to health that research on it formed the basis of the 1978 Nobel Prize in chemistry. A small number of cardiologists in the United States and Europe, and far more in Japan, have successfully used large amounts (approximately 400 mg daily) of supplemental CoQ_{10} to treat cardiomyopathy and heart failure, diseases characterized by a catastrophic loss of energy in heart cells.

All of these findings should raise red flags about the use of statins in lowering cholesterol and, now, in lowering CRP levels. One common side effect of statins is muscle weakness, which is significant because muscle cells (particularly the heart) contain the largest amounts of CoQ_{10}. In August 2001, Bayer A.G., a giant German pharmaceutical company, withdrew its Baycol statin drug from the marketplace. Thirty-one patients had died while taking the drug, all because of a rare condition in which muscle tissue broke down.

Events in 2008 further questioned the therapeutic benefits of statins. Merck and Schering-Plough Pharmaceuticals announced in a news release (not in a medical journal article) that two of their drugs, Zetia and Vytorin, lowered cholesterol levels but did *not* slow the development of artery-clogging fatty plaque. (Zetia slows the absorption of cholesterol from the gut, and Vytorin combines Zetia with Zocor, a cholesterol-lowering statin drug.) Ominously, the research suggested that Vytorin *increased* the risk of suffering a heart attack.

The announcement came after an intensive advertising campaign for Vytorin in magazines and on television. And even though the drugs did not prevent heart disease, the American Heart Association quickly issued a news release in support of the drugs. Why would the American Heart Association give credence to drugs that don't work? According to an article in the *New York Times*, the American Heart Association receives $2 million a year from the pharmaceutical collaboration of Merck and Schering-Plough Pharmaceuticals. Zetia and Vytorin earned the drug companies $5 billion in revenues in 2007 alone.

As if these negative reports weren't enough, two analyses of Vytorin data strongly suggested that the drug increases the risk of cancer. One analysis found that 102 of the patients taking Vytorin developed cancer, compared with 67 of those taking placebos. The other analysis found 93 cases of cancer among people taking Vytorin, versus 65 cases among those taking placebos.

In the next chapter and the remainder of this book, we will focus on safe dietary changes and supplements to boost the body's production of natural anti-inflammatory substances.

PART II

The AI Diet Plan

CHAPTER 6

Fourteen Steps to Fight the Inflammation Syndrome

By now, you understand how the current American (or Western-style) diet has set the stage for chronic inflammation, and you know that a permanent solution cannot be found in over-the-counter or prescription drugs. In this chapter, I describe fourteen dietary steps that will guide you toward anti-inflammatory foods and away from pro-inflammatory foods. I'll also discuss one of the side benefits of these better eating habits: if you are overweight, you will likely lose weight.

I call my dietary recommendations the AI Diet Plan. AI stands for two related concepts. One is "*anti-inflammation*," and the other is "*action item*." The AI abbreviation should help you remember that my diet steps are both anti-inflammatory *and* action items for you. The AI Diet Plan has two benefits. One, it starts to correct some of the damage that occurred during the years you followed a pro-inflammatory diet. Two, it helps you maintain a diet that reduces your future risk of developing chronic inflammation.

In practice, my AI steps are linked to one another. For example, if you adhere strictly to step 1, you won't have to memorize most of the others. And following just some of the steps most of the time should lead to a significant improvement in how you feel. Of course, you'll achieve optimal results by following all fourteen of the AI steps.

The AI Diet Plan steps are not difficult, but you may experience an initial adjustment period. The reason is that you'll be breaking the bad eating habits that made you unhealthy and replacing them with better eating habits. There is a learning curve with selecting and preparing healthier foods, just as there is when it comes to using a new computer or camera. It often helps to clean out your refrigerator and pantry to get rid of unhealthy foods. If you dread the effort or the commitment to the AI Diet Plan, I'll ask that you do your best in following some of my steps for only one week. You will likely start to feel much better during this time.

—∽—

Jack's AI Diet Steps

1. Eat a variety of fresh and whole foods.
2. Eat more fish, especially coldwater varieties.
3. Eat lean meat from free-range or grass-fed animals.
4. Eat a lot of high-fiber, nonstarchy vegetables and fruits.
5. Use more spices and herbs to flavor foods.
6. Use only healthy oils for cooking.
7. When thirsty, opt for water and other natural beverages.
8. Snack on nuts and seeds.
9. Eat organically produced foods as much as you can afford to.
10. Identify and avoid food allergens.
11. Avoid conventional cooking oils.
12. Strictly limit sugars and sugary foods.
13. Limit your intake of refined grains.
14. Consider reducing your intake of dairy foods.

—∽—

Jack's AI Step 1: Eat a Variety of Fresh and Whole Foods

Most of my anti-inflammatory dietary steps are spinoffs of this first, all-important one: eat a variety of fresh and whole foods. Fresh, whole foods are distinguished by two traits: One, they have not been processed or altered beyond refrigeration, cutting or slicing, and cooking. Two, fresh foods look something like the way they did in nature. In other words, a piece of fish looks like it came from a fish, a piece of chicken looks like it came from a chicken, and vegetables look like vegetables. Fish sticks, chicken nuggets, and onion rings don't look like anything found in nature or grown on a farm.

As a general rule, I recommend against consuming any food that bears little resemblance to what it looked like in nature. Following this principle means being circumspect about most foods sold in boxes, cans, jars, bottles, tubs, and bags. It also means dutifully reading the ingredients list on food labels. This vigilance doesn't apply only to shopping in supermarkets. It also pertains to foods sold at health food stores because some of these foods and beverages may be brimming with sugars and other processed carbohydrates. I have occasionally been stung when I neglected to follow my own advice here. For example, I once bought a bag of dried cranberries, only to find their natural tartness diluted by added sugar.

Even many natural or natural-appearing foods have undergone a fair amount of alteration or tampering. Applesauce and apple juice lack the fiber of an apple and, as a result, provide a hefty dose of sugars, which contributes to inflammation. Many brands of peanut butter contain added trans fats (in the form of partially hydrogenated vegetable oils), sugar, and salt. It defies the imagination that a snack as simple as peanut butter has so often been nutritionally perverted.

Of course, there are exceptions to this fresh-and-whole-rule, and not every packaged food is bad or unhealthy. Extra-virgin olive oil is processed and comes in bottles, but it is a healthy cooking oil. Culinary spices, such as basil, oregano, and turmeric, are processed in the sense that they are dehydrated and ground, but they are also good for you. And because I mentioned peanut butter, there are many brands of pure peanut butter at natural food stores and perhaps even a grinder to make peanut butter on the spot.

I do not consider breads and other grain-derived foods, such as pasta, bagels, and muffins, to be whole foods. The reason is that all grain products, even whole-grain varieties, undergo extensive processing and alteration. I'll address the issue of bread and grains more under AI Step 13. For now, if you avoid packaged and processed foods and grains, you are left with essentially two food groups, one consisting of quality protein (e.g., fish, chicken, or eggs) and the other consisting of vegetables and fruit. I often refer to these food groups as P and P—for protein and produce—and they form the heart of my dietary recommendations.

At this point, you may be asking yourself whether preparing mostly fresh foods means you'll have to spend an inordinate amount of time cooking. Fresh foods will take a little more time to cut and cook, compared with simply zapping a box for five minutes in a microwave oven. But fresh foods won't take a lot more time, and the recipes in this book and my other books (e.g., *Stop Prediabetes Now* and *The Food-Mood Solution*) are generally geared to quick preparation. Furthermore, you'll spend far less time shopping for foods at the supermarket, and you'll be able to avoid entire aisles there. If I may be especially blunt, you can either make the time to prepare healthy foods today—or be forced to make the time to be disabled in a few years. Given this choice, you shouldn't find it a difficult decision to begin to prepare healthier foods.

Jack's AI Step 2: Eat More Fish, Especially Coldwater Varieties

Coldwater fish, such as salmon, herring, and sardines, contain the largest amounts of the most biologically active dietary omega-3 fatty acids, specifically eicosapentaenoic acid (EPA) and docosahexaenoic acid (DHA), which I discussed in chapter 3 and will again come back to in chapter 8. Because EPA and DHA are "preformed," the body does not have to make them from alpha-linolenic acid. EPA and DHA are quickly converted to anti-inflammatory prostaglandins, such as prostaglandin E_3.

People differ in their optimal amounts of omega-3 fats. For the average healthy person, about 7 grams of omega-3s, the amount found in two to three servings of coldwater fish, is a good weekly amount. This amount translates to about 1 gram of fish oil capsules daily. People with chronic inflammatory disorders, however, will likely need much larger amounts of fish or fish oil capsules. Eating fish (e.g., salmon, herring, and sardines) three to four times a week is a good target during the first couple of months on my AI Diet Plan. Fish oil supplements, which will also be discussed in chapter 8, almost always improve the body's ability to control inflammation.

What kind of salmon should you buy? Wild salmon contains a higher portion of anti-inflammatory omega-3 fatty acids compared with farmed salmon. Farmed salmon (often sold as Atlantic salmon) are fed grains and, as a result, end up having a higher percentage of pro-inflammatory omega-6 fatty acids, although they still contain some omega-3s. Farmed salmon have another disadvantage, in that they tend to have high levels of dioxin, a cancer-causing industrial pollutant.

Unfortunately, farmed salmon tends to predominate in markets and restaurants. Pay close attention to package labels, which, by law, should identify whether the fish is wild or farmed. If you buy unlabeled fish at the counter, ask whether it is wild or farmed. All types of Alaskan salmon, including king, coho, and sockeye, are always wild. Other excellent sources of omega-3s include mackerel, anchovy, sardines, herring, and lake trout. Tuna, halibut, cod, sole, snapper, crab, and shrimp contain smaller quantities of omega-3s, but they are still healthy.

Fish is always better (and smells less "fishy") when fresh, compared with frozen and defrosted. Unfortunately, most fish is delivered frozen to supermarkets and is allowed to defrost in the "fresh fish case." You may broil, bake, poach, grill, or pan-fry the fish in olive or macadamia nut oil (and you should specify one of these cooking methods when ordering fish in restaurants). Never, ever eat breaded, deep-fried fish. The breading adds empty calories, and the frying saturates the breading and the fish with pro-inflammatory omega-6 fatty acids and trans fats.

It's more difficult to increase your dietary intake of EPA and DHA if you are a strict vegetarian, if you dislike the taste of fish, or if you are allergic to fish. Freshly ground flaxseed can be sprinkled on a salad or mixed in unsweetened yogurt, and flaxseed oil can be drizzled on cooked vegetables or used in a salad dressing. Although flax contains large amounts of alpha-linolenic acid, you may not efficiently convert it to EPA and DHA.

—⚏—

The Issue of Mercury in Fish

Many people are wary about eating fish because of the potential risk of mercury contamination; however, this issue is not as straightforward as people often think.

Smaller fish, such as sardines and anchovies, tend to be the least contaminated by mercury, mainly because they are lower on the food chain. They're also rich in omega-3s. Salmon are toward the top of the fish food chain, and because they feed on large amounts of smaller fish, they are more likely to accumulate mercury.

The toxicity of mercury is strongly influenced by your intake of dietary selenium. Selenium and mercury have a chemical affinity for each other, and toxicologists have long known that selenium binds to mercury, rendering it nontoxic. Most multivitamin/multimineral supplements provide 200 micrograms (mcg) of selenium daily; you can safely supplement up to 400 mcg daily.

If you are pregnant or planning to become pregnant, however, it may be best to err on the side of caution. Low-mercury seafood includes anchovy, crawfish, Pacific flounder, herring, king crab, sanddabs, scallops, Pacific sole, tilapia, wild Alaska and Pacific salmon, clams, striped bass, and sturgeon. If you are pregnant, you can opt for fish oil capsules, which provide the omega-3s but contain no mercury.

—ɷ—

Jack's AI Step 3: Eat Lean Meat from Free-Range or Grass-Fed Animals

Paleolithic humans and early animal herders ate meat from free-range, grass-fed animals. Grass is a rich source of alpha-linolenic acid, the parent molecule of omega-3s, which ruminants convert to EPA and DHA. When our ancestors ate the meat of these animals, they consumed large amounts of anti-inflammatory omega-3 fatty acids. Today, when farm animals eat mostly corn and other grains, their muscles contain virtually no omega-3 fatty acids. Instead, their marbled fat consists of substantial amounts of saturated fat and pro-inflammatory arachidonic acid, the hub of the omega-6s' pro-inflammatory activity.

When you follow my AI Diet Plan, it is important that you avoid or strictly limit your intake of meat from corn-fed animals. Whenever possible, opt for meat from free-range or grass-fed animals. Many natural food stores, such as Natural Grocers by Vitamin Cottage and Whole Foods, sell meat from free-range or grass-fed animals. On occasion, so does Trader Joe's. Some livestock is "finished" on grains, so meat from fully grass-fed animals is best.

Unfortunately, the choices are not as clear cut when it comes to purchasing chicken, eggs, or turkey. Whole Foods and Trader Joe's tend to sell chicken, eggs, or turkey from animals that have been given organic feed. Unfortunately, that organic feed is usually grain. On the positive side, chicken and turkey meat is generally low in fat, so they should be relatively neutral as sources of the omega-6s and the omega-3s. Whenever possible, though, try to buy chicken, turkey, and eggs from animals that were allowed to peck around for their natural diet, rather than being fed corn and other grains.

Jack's AI Step 4: Eat a Lot of High-Fiber, Nonstarchy Vegetables and Fruits

Most vegetables and fruits are the best dietary sources of antioxidants, which help dampen overactive immune responses. Contrary to popular opinion, the majority of these antioxidants are not vitamins. The lion's share belongs to a large family of vitaminlike nutrients known as polyphenolic flavonoids. More than 5,000 flavonoids (one subfamily among polyphenols) have been identified in plants. A small apple (about 3.5 ounces) contains approximately 5.7 mg of vitamin C, but more than 500 mg of antioxidant polyphenolic flavonoids, which are the antioxidant equivalent of 1,500 mg of vitamin C.

Vegetables and fruits are also rich sources of carotenoids, another class of powerful antioxidants. Although more than six hundred carotenoids have been found in nature, only a handful appear important for humans. These include alpha-carotene, beta-carotene, lutein, and lycopene.

I recommend that you eat mostly high-fiber, nonstarchy vegetables and fruits. These vegetables include almost anything you would add to a salad, such as lettuce, spinach, tomatoes, mushrooms, and cucumbers. I would also include broccoli, cauliflower, fennel (anise) bulbs, garlic, green beans, kale, leeks, mustard greens, onions, and shallots. If you are trying to lose weight, do not eat any form of potato and minimize your intake of corn.

Aim for diversity in the vegetables and the fruits you eat. Do your best to eat five to ten servings of vegetables and fruits daily, and make a point of incorporating different types into your diet. Try to have one large salad each day, with dark green leafy lettuces (not iceberg lettuce), spinach, tomatoes, scallions, shredded carrots, mushrooms, and other vegetables. You can certainly add some grilled chicken, fish, or shrimp to the salad.

Use vegetables as a side to your meat or seafood. The vegetables can be steamed, sautéed, or grilled. For example, you can steam broccoli or cauliflower one day, sauté asparagus pieces and spinach another day, and grill slices of squash, eggplant, and fennel on yet another day. Adding a small amount of garlic, olive oil, and lemon will enhance the flavor of most cooked vegetables.

Most fruits have been cultivated for a high sugar content, and I often discourage people from eating bananas and pears if they are overweight or have high blood sugar. As with vegetables, I recommend high-fiber, nonstarchy fruits, such as raspberries, blueberries, blackberries, and kiwifruit. Often, frozen berries are less expensive than fresh, but always check bags of frozen fruit to ensure that no sugars have been added. Canned fruit almost always contains added sugars.

Jack's AI Step 5: Use More Spices and Herbs to Flavor Foods

The omnipresent salt and pepper shakers in homes and restaurants reflect both an excess of dietary sodium and a lack of more interesting—and anti-inflammatory—herbs and spices in the average American diet.

In ancient times, the human diet provided large amounts of potassium and small amounts of naturally occurring sodium. Today's meals contain substantial quantities of salt, some of it added during the manufacture of food products and often still more added at the table. As a result, our meals typically contain far more sodium than potassium. This alters the body's acid-alkaline balance, leading to lower bone density and increased muscle loss. An altered acid-alkaline balance may even influence the risk of developing chronic inflammation.

Salt is best used in moderation. (Celtic Sea Salt and RealSalt are good brands of salt that are not overly processed.) As an alternative, I recommend emphasizing a variety of culinary spices and herbs to create exciting new flavors and to keep foods from becoming boring. Basil, oregano, and garlic are a wonderful combination. So are garlic and rosemary, garlic and saffron, and Indian curry blends (including turmeric, coriander, cardamom, cayenne, and cumin). The benefits of these spices go beyond their taste. These and other herbs and spices are rich in antioxidants and Cox-2 inhibitors. They may not by themselves have the effect of aspirin or prescription pain relievers, but they can enhance the benefits of an anti-inflammatory diet.

Jack's AI Step 6: Use Only Healthy Oils for Cooking

I recommend that extra-virgin olive oil be your primary cooking oil. It's healthy and easy to find at markets. Extra-virgin olive oil is made from the first pressing of olives. Any olive oil that is not labeled "extra virgin" has undergone subsequent processing. Two other cooking oils are just as good, however, and have different advantages, in that their flavor is more neutral and they can be used at higher temperatures. They are macadamia nut oil and avocado oil.

All three oils are rich in anti-inflammatory oleic acid (an omega-9 fatty acid), vitamin E, and polyphenolic flavonoids. Olive oils often have stronger flavors and a greater variety in flavors. For example, Greek Kalamata olive oil has a rich, thicker flavor, whereas most Italian, Spanish, and California olive oils tend to have a lighter flavor. I sometimes cook with Kalamata olive oil but will always use a lighter olive oil as a salad dressing.

Macadamia nut oil is also rich in oleic acid, the same anti-inflammatory omega-9 fatty acid found in olive oil. I find macadamia nut oil particularly nice when I'm cooking Indian or Asian meals and don't want the Mediterranean flavor of olive oil. My favorite brand is Australian MacNut oil. (See www.mac-nut-oil.com.) If it is pricey, however, you may be able to find less expensive brands at natural food stores.

I recently discovered a line of high-quality avocado cooking oils, which are also rich in oleic acid. Pure avocado oil has a neutral flavor that, again, works well in both Mediterranean-style and other cuisines, such as Asian and Indian. In addition, the marketer of these oils, Olivado, sells several other varieties of avocado oil infused with basil, lemon, rosemary, or chile. These oils can be used in both cooking and as oil-and-vinegar salad dressings. (See www.olivado.com.)

Although our Paleolithic ancestors did not consume any kind of pressed oil, these oils are an acceptable compromise for our modern eating habits. The omega-9 fatty acids work synergistically with the omega-3s. In addition, a small amount of butter, used with olive or macadamia nut oils, adds a nice flavor when sautéing fish or chicken.

Don't ever heat fish oil or flaxseed oil, and don't use them as cooking oils. High temperatures rapidly oxidize and break them down, leading to the formation of pro-inflammatory free radicals. It is fine, of course, to cook fish because its protein and water content resist those high temperatures, unless, of course, you happen to overcook or burn it.

Jack's AI Step 7: When Thirsty, Opt for Water and Other Natural Beverages

Many people have difficulty giving up soft drinks for simple water, a beverage that is often perceived as boring and tasteless. Yet water is part of our biological heritage. All animals consume water throughout their lives, except for mammals that breast-feed during infancy. Humans are the only animal that intentionally consumes liquids besides water and mother's milk.

The widespread use of bottled water does reflect a positive shift away from soft drinks, although plastic bottles (which are not always recycled) create an enormous amount of waste. If the taste of tap water does not appeal to you, or if you are concerned about chlorine or contaminants, consider using a filtration system. The simplest systems consist of water pitchers with filters, such as those made by Brita and Pur. Some water-filtering systems attach to kitchen faucets. Brita and Pur filters remove chlorine, heavy metals, and undesirable compounds. With filtered water, you can easily refill an environmentally friendly stainless-steel or plastic bottle and carry it with you while commuting.

There are many ways to give water an interesting and tasty twist. Perrier, San Pellegrino, Gerolsteiner, Blu, and other brands of European sparkling mineral water contain respectable amounts of calcium, magnesium, and other nutrients. If you find that mineral waters taste flat, add a wedge of lemon, lime, or orange. Consider as well two brands of flavored waters that contain a hint of fruit or vegetable flavor. Both Hint (www.drinkhint.com) and Ayala (www.herbalwater.com) waters are tasty and do not contain calories, sugars, or artificial sweeteners. My personal favorites are Hint's Lime, Raspberry-Lime, and Pomegranate-Tangerine flavors, and Ayala's Ginger-Lime Peel, Cinnamon-Orange Peel, and Cloves-Cardamom-Cinnamon flavors. Hint and Ayala are available at many natural food markets.

It is also easy to make iced tea by adding a teabag or two to a pitcher of room-temperature water and allowing it to steep for one hour before refrigerating. You can use conventional black teas, which provide substantial amounts of antioxidant nutrients. My favorite iced tea is a green tea that goes by the not-very-catchy name of Catechin-Rich Tea. (Catechins are a type of antioxidant found in tea.) One teabag of Catechin-Rich Tea (www.miroku-usa.com) makes a full pitcher in fifteen minutes and tastes better than any other iced green tea I've had.

I recently discovered coconut water, a common beverage in South America, the Caribbean islands, and Asia. It is now available in the United States and is sold in recyclable packages that preserve its flavor and protect against bacterial contamination. Coconut water is often recommended as a rehydrating drink after exercise: an 11-ounce serving provides approximately 660 mg of potassium, along with small amounts of calcium, magnesium, and sodium. An 11-ounce serving of coconut water also contains approximately 60 calories and 14 grams of carbohydrates, most in the form of naturally occurring sugars, roughly one-third the calories and carbohydrates found in the same amount of a soft drink. Despite the calories, coconut water is one of the healthiest beverages.

—ᗰ—

Navigating Restaurant Menus

At home, you can control what you eat. Step into a restaurant, however, and you enter a nutritional minefield. Fast-food restaurants (e.g., McDonald's, Burger King, and KFC) are the worst, serving up meal after meal built around refined carbohydrates, sugars, omega-6 fats, and trans fats. Although you may enter one of these restaurants with good intentions, the smell of fries may weaken your willpower. And even if all you want is a salad, you will likely be sabotaged by a salad dressing that uses soybean oil (instead of olive oil).

Some national chains, such as Denny's and IHOP, aren't much better, but it is possible to navigate their menus. You can order a burger or a chicken (not breaded and deep-fried) sandwich, minus the bun. Ask for steamed vegetables, such as broccoli, or a small salad instead of fries. A chef's salad is another safe option, but always order salads with an oil-and-vinegar dressing.

Restaurants that serve fresh fish (e.g., McCormick and Schmick's) are a good bet, although they can be pricier than other types of restaurants. Greek, Italian, and Middle Eastern restaurants are fairly easy to navigate, as long as you avoid the ever-present pita breads, rice, pasta, and deep-fried food (e.g., falafel). These cuisines use olive oil almost exclusively. In a Japanese restaurant, you can order salmon teriyaki—but ask that the chef squeeze some lemon on the fish instead of using the sugary teriyaki sauce. If you like raw fish, order the sashimi. (Sushi comes with white rice; sashimi does not.) Although buckwheat noodles are starchy, they're made from the seed of a fruit, not from any type of wheat. Mexican restaurants tend to be heavy on wheat, corn, and dairy. You're better off eating fajitas, but skip the tortilla, rice, and beans.

—ᗰ—

Jack's AI Step 8: Snack on Nuts and Seeds

Most people like to snack or indulge their sweet tooth. A nutritionally safe approach is to make your own trail mix from raw, unsalted almonds, cashews, filberts, macadamias, pistachios, and pumpkin seeds. You can buy these nuts and seeds in bags or in the bulk section of some markets. Mix them together in a large bowl, then transfer them to small plastic bags you can keep in your purse, desk, or car.

Nuts and seeds are both relatively high in linoleic acid, an acceptable source of omega-6 fatty acids, and the fat gives them a sweet taste. Another option is almond butter, which has a natural sweetness and is less allergenic than peanuts.

Many studies have found that eating nuts (preferably those that are raw or unsalted) reduces the risk of developing heart disease. This benefit may be related to the amount of magnesium and other minerals found in nuts and seeds.

Jack's AI Step 9: Eat Organically Produced Foods as Much as You Can Afford To

Organic foods are produced without synthetic pesticides in an environmentally sustainable fashion. This means that the soil quality (nitrogen and mineral content) is preserved and enhanced, which is different from the way conventional farming practices tend to drain and not replenish nutrients.

Organics provide clear benefits for you. One is that they are free of pesticides and genetically engineered material. Many pesticides are estrogen mimics, meaning that they simulate the effect of estrogen and may disrupt the activities of your own hormones. Although the connection between pesticides and inflammation is tenuous, there is a clear link between pesticides and certain diseases, such as cancer and Parkinson's disease, which do have inflammatory underpinnings. In any event, it is smart to minimize your exposure to pesticides.

The second justification is that several research studies have found that organically raised vegetables and fruits tend to contain higher vitamin and mineral levels, compared with conventionally grown produce. And, although this is a subjective judgment, many people say that organics taste better than conventional vegetables and fruit. You don't have to be an expert to taste the difference between a supermarket tomato and an organic one from a local farmer's market.

When it comes to meat, try to buy cuts from free-range or grass-fed animals. These two choices are likely to be pesticide free and also relatively high in anti-inflammatory omega-3 fatty acids. Often, "organically raised" chicken and beef are from animals fed organic grains that, organic or not, are high in pro-inflammatory omega-6 fatty acids. Those omega-6 fatty acids are incorporated into the animals' fat and ultimately into yours.

Unfortunately, organic produce and meat from free-range or grass-fed animals cost more than conventionally produced foods. The difference in cost is related mostly to economies of scale—organic producers tend to be smaller operations, whereas conventional producers tend to be very large, streamlined businesses. I am also sensitive to the fact that many people (including me) simply cannot afford to eat organic foods all the time. My advice is to buy what you can comfortably afford; you may find the best bargains at farmers' markets, not at natural food stores. If you can't afford organic foods, just follow as many of my other AI Diet Plan steps as possible.

Jack's AI Step 10: Identify and Avoid Food Allergens

Food allergies and allergylike food sensitivities rev up the immune system and promote either acute or chronic low-grade inflammation. It is relatively easy to obtain a "food allergy panel," based on a blood test, from a nutritionally oriented physician. Some supermarkets even sponsor healthmobiles that can perform rudimentary allergy test panels for $30 to $50. These panels test people's reactions to a variety of foods.

If you pay attention to your own responses to food, you may be able to accurately self-diagnose food sensitivities. Wheat, dairy, and soy are the most common food sensitivities, but people can be sensitive to any type of healthy or junk food. (Sharp fluctuations in blood sugar may also be intertwined with food sensitivities and may affect your reactions to food.) Some people have obvious allergic reactions to foods, such as developing hives after eating shrimp or strawberries. Other reactions may be subtle; for example, you develop the sniffles or get drowsy after eating a certain food. Food allergies can also take the form of a food addiction, and to self-diagnose this type of sensitivity, simply think about the foods you really love, crave, or can't imagine living without. People often tell me how important coffee, chocolate, and bread are to them—and I immediately suspect food addictions and sensitivities.

If you suspect that you have food sensitivities, keep a diary of how you react after eating, and then try to correlate the changes in how you feel (physically and emotionally) to specific foods. Another option is to avoid all foods belonging to a particular family (such as all dairy products) for a week. You may notice that you feel better by the end of the week. Whether you do or don't feel better, reintroduce foods from that family (e.g., milk, cream, or cheese). If you suddenly feel worse, you are likely sensitive to that food.

Gluten sensitivity often falls within the realm of food sensitivity, although the biochemical mechanism is different from other types of food reactions. Gluten refers to a family of proteins found in wheat, rye, and barley. The most severe form of gluten intolerance is usually diagnosed as celiac disease, which affects roughly one in every hundred people. In celiac disease, an immune response destroys part of the intestinal wall, which can affect bowel habits and nutrient absorption, leading to secondary nutritional deficiencies. Because celiac disease can interfere with iron and calcium absorption, anemia and osteoporosis are common consequences. Some experts believe that lesser degrees of gluten intolerance may affect one of every two people. Many of the people who are gluten sensitive also react to casein, which is a problem in dairy products.

Nightshades are another problematic group of foods for many people, particularly those with rheumatoid arthritis. The late nutritionist and public health educator Carlton Fredericks, Ph.D., noted that one of every five people with rheumatoid arthritis was sensitive to nightshades. This family of plants includes tomatoes, potatoes, eggplants, and bell and chile peppers. Tobacco is also a member of the nightshade family. Before Columbus noticed Native Americans eating tomatoes and peppers, Europeans thought that all nightshades were poisonous. Given the prevalence of tomatoes and potatoes in meals (including ketchup on fries), it is advisable for people with arthritis to avoid these foods for several weeks to see whether their symptoms decrease.

—ɯ—

Navigating the Supermarket

To improve your odds of buying healthier foods, shop mostly along the store's perimeter. This applies to both supermarkets and natural food stores, because nearly all markets follow a similar floor plan, with refrigerated foods (produce, meat, seafood, and dairy) on the perimeter. Most fresh foods require refrigeration, and you'll want to do most of your food shopping in the produce, meat, and fish departments.

As you move toward the center of the store, you will find entire aisles devoted to soft drinks, cookies, breads, and cereals. These foods are incompatible with the AI Diet Plan. The same is largely true for the frozen-food aisles. Although you should be able to find bags of frozen vegetables (without anything added), the freezers typically contain mostly highly processed microwave meals, ice cream, and high-sugar juices.

You'll find that the AI Diet Plan will actually simplify and speed the time you spend shopping. That's because you'll be able to ignore most of the supermarket aisles.

—⚭—

Jack's AI Step 11: Avoid Conventional Cooking Oils

Olive, macadamia nut, sesame, walnut, and coconut and avocado oils and a little butter are fine (see Jack's AI Step 6), but I recommend throwing out any bottles of corn, soybean, peanut, safflower, sunflower, canola, and cottonseed oils you might have in your kitchen. (You can do this as part of a general pantry cleanup to dispose of unhealthy foods.) These processed cooking oils are high in pro-inflammatory omega-6 fatty acids, and they are also found in many processed and packaged foods, including microwave meals, breakfast bars, and salad dressings. In fact, the virtual omnipresence of these oils is largely why the contemporary Western diet contains twenty to thirty times more pro-inflammatory than anti-inflammatory oils.

Partially hydrogenated vegetable oils, which contain trans fats, are among the worst of these oils because they alter how your body processes fats. Vegetable shortenings and hard margarines are common sources of partially hydrogenated vegetable oils and trans fats, but you will also likely find them in fried foods, salad dressings, nondairy creamers, and bakery products (e.g., doughnuts, cookies, and cakes). Even foods that claim to have zero trans fats may still contain some, if the ingredients include any kind of partially hydrogenated oil.

Although fast-food restaurants have claimed to reduce or eliminate trans fats, they continue to give customers a hefty dose of these unhealthy oils. For example, McDonald's currently claims that its fries and chicken nuggets have no trans fats, but the restaurant's burgers and dessert items contain substantial amounts of trans fats. Likewise, trans fats are still a common ingredient in many KFC meals, and the restaurant's Chicken and Biscuit Bowl contains a whopping 4.5 grams of trans fats, according to www.kfc.com.

Many fast-food restaurants are switching from partially hydrogenated vegetable oils (i.e., trans fats) to interesterified fats. Like hydrogenation, interesterification is another way of processing fats, but a study found that interesterified fats dangerously increased blood sugar levels in only one month. Perhaps worse, some types of interesterified fats also contain trans fats. Interesterified fats may be listed by that term or as fully hydrogenated or hydrogenated vegetable oils on package labels. Fast-food meals do not typically come with ingredient lists, however (although nutrition information is available at fast-food Web sites).

Cooking oils that are rich in processed omega-6 fatty acids, trans fats, and interesterified fats are dangerous and either directly or indirectly pro-inflammatory. My best advice is to avoid any food package or restaurant meal that uses any cooking oil other than olive oil or macadamia nut oil.

Jack's AI Step 12: Strictly Limit Sugars and Sugary Foods

Refined sugars are the ultimate empty calories, devoid of any necessary nutrition. In many respects, they are actually *anti*-nutrients because they deplete the levels of certain vitamins (particularly vitamin B_1) that are needed to metabolize them. The consumption of sugars and sugarlike carbohydrates (white breads, muffins, pasta, bagels) increases levels of C-reactive protein, a marker and promoter of inflammation.

Added sugars are omnipresent in processed and packaged foods. The most common types are listed as sucrose, high-fructose corn syrup, dextrose, glucose, fructose, and corn syrup. Most boxes of salt contain a little sugar, and some sugar substitutes (particularly, NutraSweet and Equal) contain some sugar in the form of maltodextrose.

With two-thirds of Americans now overweight or obese, there are no nutritional justifications for people to consume large quantities of sugars—now, an average of 150 pounds annually for every man, woman, and child in the United States. Some athletes, such as cyclists, believe they need sugary gels, drinks, and bars to sustain their energy, but fruit can provide the same benefits, along with important vitamins and minerals.

Various types of sweets (including breakfast bars, sweetened coffee drinks, and desserts), soft drinks, and fruit juices are the principal sources of dietary sugars. Vast numbers of packaged foods, however, contain small amounts of sugar that do add up. Sixty years ago, most soft drinks were sold in small 6-ounce bottles. Today, cans of soft drinks double that amount. A half-gallon (64-ounce) soft drink bottle contains approximately *one-half pound* of sugar, some a little less and others a little more. Convenience and large quantities breed overconsumption.

Healthy-appearing fruit juices can be deceiving and even worse than soft drinks. For example, a two-quart bottle of Ocean Spray Cranberry Juice Cocktail contains 1,040 calories, more than a half-pound of sugar (264 grams)—and nearly all of it comes from high-fructose corn syrup. A two-quart bottle of Welch's 100% Grape Juice contains 1,360 calories and almost three-quarters of a pound (320 grams) of sugar. It doesn't matter whether these are natural or added sugars—they come with virtually no other nutritional value.

"Raw sugar" might sound healthier, but it is merely dirty white sugar that contains almost undetectable amounts of a few minerals (which can be obtained in far greater amounts in other, more nutritious, foods). An occasional little bit of honey is acceptable—it is far too sweet to consume in excess. My favorite natural sweetener is stevia, made from an herbal leaf, which is three hundred times sweeter than sugar. Adding a few stevia drops to beverages works fine, but be wary of stevia powders, some of which are mixed with lactose, a milk sugar. If you have frequent or intense sugar cravings, consider the possibility that you may have prediabetes or type 2 diabetes. My book *Stop Prediabetes Now* discusses those issues in depth.

Jack's AI Step 13: Limit Your Intake of Refined Grains

Like sugars, refined-grain products (e.g., breads, cereals, and pastas) provide mostly empty calories, even though many of these foods have been "enriched" with a few vitamins. The reality is that scores of nutrients have been removed through processing, refining, and bleaching, leaving mostly starch. Many processed foods contain a combination of what I consider an unholy nutritional trinity: refined grains, sugars, and partially hydrogenated vegetable oils. I refer to these grain-based products as being sugarlike carbohydrates because their effect on blood sugar and C-reactive protein is so similar to that of pure sugars.

Wheat is the most common grain in most Western diets, but corn and rice are also problematic. Both wheat and rice contain lectins, a family of proteins that interferes with the absorption of vitamins and minerals. Some research indicates that lectins may trigger an abnormal immune response and may also be a factor in rheumatoid arthritis.

Whole grains (e.g., whole-wheat or multigrain bread) have few advantages over refined grains (e.g., white bread). Whole grains do contain a few more vitamins and minerals and more fiber, but they are still major sources of starch that a predominantly overweight population really doesn't need. The truth is that grain products are a relatively recent addition to the human diet, and people may not be genetically adapted to consuming grains. In addition, human teeth cannot chew grain seeds, and even whole-grain breads would not be possible without processing. When grains (e.g., wheat and rye) are ground into flour, they have more of a sugarlike effect on blood sugar, which can contribute to both prediabetes and inflammation.

You may not have to avoid all grains while on the AI Diet Plan. If your weight and blood sugar are normal, and if you are gluten tolerant, you can eat some grain products. I view them as an occasional treat, and I limit my intake. I consume small amounts of brown, purple, and red rice varieties (see www.lotusfoods.com for more information). I never eat cereal, and I rarely buy any bread or wheat or corn flour to use at home.

—⚬—

Smoking and Inflammation

Tobacco is highly addictive, and almost everyone who smokes (or chews) tobacco products knows that these are harmful. In addition to increasing the risk of lung cancer, tobacco smoke raises the odds of developing other types of cancer, emphysema, and coronary artery disease. Smoking also elevates levels of C-reactive protein, a powerful promoter of inflammation. Even after a person stops smoking, his or her CRP levels remain higher than normal for years. So if you don't smoke, don't even think of starting. And if you do smoke, please try to break the habit.

—⚬—

Jack's AI Step 14: Consider Reducing Your Intake of Dairy Foods

Like grains, dairy products are a relatively recent addition to the human diet, and some scientific research suggests that adults would do better limiting their intake of most dairy products, such as milk, cream, cheese, ice cream, and yogurt. Dairy products are one of the most common food allergens, although people tend to react less frequently to yogurt and hard cheeses, most likely because bacteria have predigested much of the protein.

Many people, particularly Asians and Africans, lose the ability to digest milk after childhood. In addition, no species (other than humans) naturally consumes the milk of another species. Cow's milk is intended to nurture calves, not humans, just as human mother's milk is meant only for human babies.

If you are not dairy sensitive, adding small amounts of hard cheese and a little unsweetened yogurt to your diet should be fine. Soft cheeses (e.g., American cheese) are processed and may contain a variety of additives. In fast-food restaurants, cheese (e.g., the cheese added to burgers) may contain partially hydrogenated vegetable oils.

You Will Likely Lose Weight Following Jack's AI Diet Plan

Three of every four Americans are now overweight, and one of every two overweight Americans is obese, weighing at least 30 pounds more than his or her ideal weight. In 2008, researchers calculated that if current trends continue, 86 percent of Americans will be overweight or obese by 2030. The prevalence of overweight and obesity is increasing around the world, typically following the increased consumption of American-style fast foods and soft drinks. The World Health Organization recently reported that overweight and obesity is now a far greater problem than starvation. More than 1.7 billion people are overweight or obese, almost three times more than the estimated 600 million undernourished people.

Being overweight, especially if some of the excess fat is around your belly, increases the likelihood of your suffering from inflammation and inflammatory diseases. There are several reasons for this. One is that fat cells secrete large amounts of two powerful inflammation-causing substances, interleukin-6 (IL-6) and C-reactive protein (CRP). Another reason is that abdominal fat cells attract white blood cells, which intermingle and also secrete IL-6 and CRP. Yet another reason is that the same eating habits that encourage weight gain—that is, consuming foods that contain trans fats, processed omega-6 fatty acids, sugars, and sugarlike carbohydrates—also promote inflammation. This is part of the reason that people who are overweight or have heart disease or diabetes typically have elevated CRP levels.

There is good news: If you are overweight and start to follow my AI Diet Plan, you will likely lose weight and your IL-6 and CRP levels will likely decline.

The AI Diet Plan emphasizes two food groups: (1) quality protein and (2) high-fiber, nonstarchy vegetables and fruits. Both protein and fiber help stabilize blood sugar and insulin, which reduces hunger, leading to

The AI Diet Plan Food Pyramid

Because of the widespread use of the U.S. Department of Agriculture's food pyramid, this drawing might help some people visualize the AI Diet Plan Pyramid. Foods toward the top are those you would eat the least of, whereas those toward the bottom are those you would eat the most of.

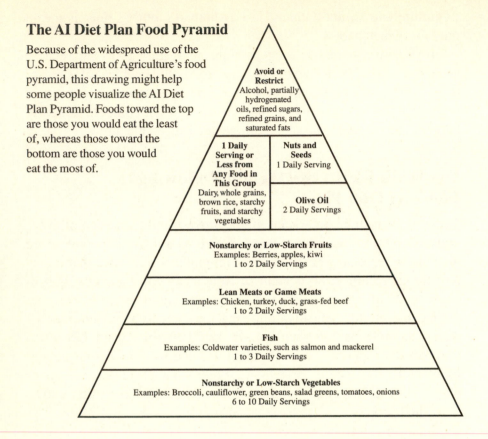

Avoid or Restrict
Alcohol, partially hydrogenated oils, refined sugars, refined grains, and saturated fats

1 Daily Serving or Less from Any Food in This Group
Dairy, whole grains, brown rice, starchy fruits, and starchy vegetables

Nuts and Seeds
1 Daily Serving

Olive Oil
2 Daily Servings

Nonstarchy or Low-Starch Fruits
Examples: Berries, apples, kiwi
1 to 2 Daily Servings

Lean Meats or Game Meats
Examples: Chicken, turkey, duck, grass-fed beef
1 to 2 Daily Servings

Fish
Examples: Coldwater varieties, such as salmon and mackerel
1 to 3 Daily Servings

Nonstarchy or Low-Starch Vegetables
Examples: Broccoli, cauliflower, green beans, salad greens, tomatoes, onions
6 to 10 Daily Servings

the consumption of less food. There is also research suggesting that the omega-3 and omega-9 fatty acids contribute to weight loss (despite their own calories).

Although you might think that my AI Diet Plan sounds a lot like the Atkins diet, it's different. I describe the AI Diet Plan as being *protein rich*, not high protein. It also contains more vegetable fiber than the Atkins diet does. The AI Diet Plan emphasizes *nutrient-dense* foods, meaning that you get a high concentration of nutrients in relatively few calories and carbohydrates. Not surprisingly, the AI Diet Plan is also a low-carb diet—grain-based carbs (again, breads, cereals, pastas) have poor nutrient density.

There's another bonus: when people increase their protein and cut back on carbohydrates, they also gain more energy. The higher energy levels are related to more stable blood sugar levels and to a reduction in inflammation. Mediators of inflammation, such as IL-6 and CRP and related compounds, often leave people feeling wiped out.

CHAPTER 7

The AI Diet Menu Plans and Recipes

By following most or all of the anti-inflammation dietary steps, you will find that it is relatively easy to order healthy meals in many restaurants. You may be wondering about what to cook at home, though. This chapter offers recipes for breakfast, lunch, and dinner, as well as a sample fourteen-day menu plan. This menu plan is merely a guideline and is not meant as a strict rule for what you must eat on any given day. Overall, this chapter takes a very positive approach to food selection, emphasizing what you should eat instead of what you should not.

Unlike many diet plans that are extremely rigid, the AI Diet Plan encourages flexibility and creativity in cooking and food choices. Inflexible dietary regimens can, for many people, become difficult to follow, and such plans often beg to be violated. So, in following the recipes in this chapter, please feel comfortable adjusting quantities, particularly of spices, to suit your personal tastes.

It is worthwhile to keep several guidelines in mind when you prepare anti-inflammatory meals at home.

1. *Healthy meals usually require some planning.* When we don't plan our meals, we tend to get distracted by deadlines, errands, or other stresses and either delay or skip meals. That leads to a blood sugar crash, and eating some type of junk food or fast food is usually the fastest, but least healthy, way to boost blood sugar. Junk foods and

fast foods tend to be high in pro-inflammatory food ingredients. Meal planning can actually be easy; simply keep a pen and a pad handy when you're watching television or driving (but make sure you've stopped before adding items to your grocery list). You can stimulate your culinary creativity by looking at recipes online or thumbing through cookbooks in bookstores.

2. *Keep your meals simple.* Many recipes are extraordinarily complex and time consuming, and few of us can prepare such meals except perhaps on weekends. I've tried to keep the recipes in this chapter relatively simple. Still, many people tell me they just don't have time to cook from scratch. But as with everything else in life, you are faced with choices: Do you want to continue living the way that made you sick, or do you want to take the steps that are necessary for you to be healthy? And do you want to take the time to cook today, or do you want to be forced to make the time to be disabled in a few years?

3. *Get a return on your investment.* Preparing food takes a bit longer than simply microwaving a frozen dinner, but investing just a few extra minutes can save a lot of time in subsequent meal preparation. It's easy to scale up (e.g., to double or triple) the quantities so that you have great-tasting leftovers. Leftovers have gotten a bad reputation—often deserved—because reheated junk foods usually taste awful. If you use quality ingredients, however, leftovers taste just as good as the original meal. A friend refers to them as "planovers." For example, leftover chicken or turkey can be diced up and scrambled with eggs for breakfast, or it can be part of a brown-bag lunch.

4. *Get creative.* There's a lot of flexibility in most recipes and methods of cooking. If you like garlic and spices, add more than the recipe calls for. If you don't like them, add less. Cooking can be a fun improv, with you modifying ingredients on the fly. If this sounds a little scary and uncertain, rest assured. I learned how to cook at age forty-nine, and I've had only a couple of really awful failures in the kitchen. Cutting and chopping up food can be meditative (although you should always keep your eye on the knife and where your fingers are), and the process of cooking is one of the most creative of all experiences. Besides, you get to eat what you have created. You can't do that with a painting.

5. *Stimulate your creative juices.* You don't have to be a "foodie," but watching the Food Network (www.foodtv.com) on television is a great way to learn cooking techniques and recipes. You can also find healthy substitutes, such as red or purple rice flours (www.lotusfoods.com) for dredging chicken and fish and to thicken sauces.

The AI Diet Plan Meals

The recipes are organized counterintuitively, with dinner first, followed by dinner side dishes, and then by lunch and breakfast. There is a reason for this type of flow. Dinner leftovers, used creatively, can become ingredients in lunches and breakfasts, thus saving you considerable time in preparing other meals. All of these recipes can be easily doubled, so that you have plenty of tasty leftovers.

—⨍—

Quick Tip: Natural Flavor Enhancers

To enhance the flavor of almost any fish or fowl, add some olive oil, garlic, or fresh-squeezed lemon juice. Oregano and basil also provide a lot of flavor, as long as they do not compete with other spices and herbs (such as herbes de Provence or dill).

—⨍—

Dinner Main Courses

Many of my anti-inflammatory recipes use salmon and other types of fish, in large part because they provide a natural source of omega-3 fats. There is also some evidence that the protein of fish is healthier than that of land animals.

Poached Salmon in Garlic-Infused Olive Oil (Serves 2)

3 to 4 garlic bulbs
olive oil, approximately 1 quart
fresh minced rosemary, about 1 tablespoon
2 skinless salmon fillets

This meal is not as oily as you might think, mainly because the oil of the salmon blocks the olive oil. First, prepare the garlic-infused olive oil. Separate the garlic cloves from the bulbs and remove the skins from the cloves. Place the cloves in a large skillet and pour in enough olive oil to cover the cloves. Bring the olive oil to a light boil, then reduce the heat, cover, and simmer for 1 to 2 hours. Using a strainer, remove the garlic and refrigerate half of it, using it later as a spread on vegetables, fish, or chicken. Next, add the rosemary and bring the oil to a light boil again for about 10 minutes. Place the salmon fillets in the oil and poach them for approximately 8 minutes per side. Remove them from the oil and serve.

(*Adapted from Devon Boisen*)

Baked Salmon (*Serves 2*)

olive oil
2 salmon fillets, about 4 to 6 ounces each
basil, to taste
oregano, to taste
1 to 3 teaspoons balsamic vinaigrette, to taste

Preheat the oven to 350 degrees F.

Coat the bottom of a baking dish with olive oil. Rinse and pat the excess water off the salmon, and place the fillets in the baking dish. Apply a thin coat of olive oil on top of them (to add flavor and to prevent burning). Sprinkle basil and oregano on the fillets. Drizzle the balsamic vinaigrette on the fillets. Bake for approximately 10 minutes. The cooking time may vary by a couple of minutes, depending on the oven and the thickness of the fillets, so examine them after 8 minutes to ensure that they are not burning or undercooked. The Baked Salmon goes well with the Spinach and Leek Sauté (page 108) and the Flavorful Brown Rice (page 109).

Pumpkin Seed–Crusted Halibut (*Serves 2*)

½ teaspoon coriander
¼ cup chopped raw pumpkin seeds
¼ cup olive oil
1 pound halibut fillet, cut into two pieces
2 pats butter
1 lemon
1 tablespoon chopped parsley

Preheat the oven to 350 degrees F.

Add the coriander to the pumpkin seeds, then chop the seeds in a food processor, being careful to avoid a flourlike texture. Meanwhile, spread the olive oil over the bottom of a baking dish. Dredge the halibut through the olive oil so that all sides of the fish are lightly coated. With one hand, spoon the chopped pumpkin seeds onto all sides of the fish, while using the fingers of your other hand to pat the seeds onto the fish. Add one pat of butter to the top of each piece of fish. Bake the fish 10 minutes per inch of thickness. When it's done, squeeze lemon juice on each piece of fish and sprinkle with parsley.

—ᴚ—

Quick Tip: Sanitary Gloves

Preparing food can often get a little messy. To avoid having to repeatedly wash your hands (such as after handling fish or rubbing olive oil into fish or meats), wear disposable, sanitary plastic gloves. Large quantities of these gloves are available inexpensively at many stores. Using these gloves also reduces possible bacterial contamination of your hands and the food.

—ᴚ—

Pan-Fried Swordfish with Citrus Marinade (*Serves 2*)

> 2 swordfish steaks, approximately 1 pound total
> 2 tablespoons olive oil
>
> **Marinade**
> 1 tablespoon olive oil
> 2 scallions, diced
> juice of 1 large lemon
> juice of 1 lime
> juice of ½ orange (optional)
> 4 cloves garlic, minced
> 1 teaspoon ground coriander
> ⅛ teaspoon cumin

Prepare the marinade by mixing the marinade ingredients in a bowl.

Trim the skin from the swordfish and soak the fish in the marinade, refrigerating it for 1 to 2 hours. When you're ready to cook, drain off as much liquid as possible from the marinade. Heat a skillet with olive oil on medium heat, then add the swordfish and the remainder of the marinade.

Cook it approximately 3 minutes per side. Serve the fish with vegetables and rice.

Roasted Salmon *(Serves 2)*

> 2 salmon fillets, with skin on one side of each fillet
> 1 tablespoon olive oil
>
> **Sauce** (2 options)
> juice of ½ lemon
> ½ stick butter, melted
>   or
> ¼ cup warm olive oil
> fresh minced garlic
> fresh minced rosemary

It might seem incongruous to roast something like fish, which is often valued for being moist rather than dried out. But roasting fish the right way—that is, quickly—should retain the moisture but give the exterior of the fish a tasty brown crust. By the way, roasting generally refers to baking above 400 degrees F (204 degrees C).

In an ovenproof pan over high heat, add the olive oil and sear the salmon fillets skin side up. Turn over the fillets, then place them in the oven at 450 degrees F for approximately 7 minutes. (The time will vary by a minute or two, depending on the thickness of the fish.) To make the sauce, mix all of the ingredients in a bowl. Spoon the sauce on the fish as soon as it comes out of the oven. You can also prepare halibut or cod this way.

(Adapted from T. Susan Chang)

Simple Poached Salmon *(Serves 4)*

> 1 quart water
> 1 cup vermouth
> 1 onion, sliced
> 1 carrot, sliced
> 1 stalk celery, sliced
> 1 bay leaf
> 1 teaspoon RealSalt, Celtic Sea Salt, or regular sea salt

1 pinch of ground black pepper
1 large fillet of salmon with skin
1 lemon

Fill a large, wide pot with water. Add the vermouth, onion, carrot, celery, bay leaf, salt, and pepper. Bring it to a boil, then simmer for 20 minutes. Meanwhile, completely wrap the salmon in a strip of cheesecloth. Fold the cheesecloth so you can unwrap it slightly to check the fish, and leave the ends long enough to drape over the sides of the pan.

Insert the fish into the simmering broth, ideally with 1 or 2 inches of water above it. Be careful to keep the ends of the cheesecloth away from the flame or heating element. Bring the water to a boil again, then simmer. Allow 8 minutes per pound for the fish to cook. Unwrap the fish to test with a fork whether it is flaky and done. If it is not done, simmer for a couple more minutes and check again.

When the fish is cooked, lift it out of the pot by grabbing it with the two ends of the cheesecloth. Place the fish on a platter and remove the cheesecloth. Squeeze lemon juice on the fish for additional flavor. The fish can be eaten with a Greek-style tzatziki cucumber-yogurt sauce (available at many supermarkets or ethnic grocers) or a mayonnaise-based sauce (find one at a natural foods grocer), along with vegetables and rice.

Baked Shrimp and Scallops (*Serves 2*)

olive oil
4 to 6 garlic cloves, diced
2 scallions, diced
12 large shrimp, peeled and cleaned
8 large scallops, sliced in half
1 teaspoon each Deliciously Dill spice mix (sold under the Spice
    Hunter label) or oregano and basil
juice of 1 lemon

Coat a large nonstick skillet or wok with olive oil. Sauté the garlic and scallions. When the scallions soften, add the shrimp, scallops, and spices. (The scallops should be sliced in half so that they cook at the same rate as the shrimp.) Add the lemon juice to create a flavorful sauce. The shrimp are cooked when they turn pink on all sides. Serve with rice and vegetables, or toss with baked spaghetti squash.

Wonderful Baked Chicken Breasts (*Serves 2*)

1 whole or 2 halves boneless and skinless chicken breasts
1 cup chicken broth
½ cup olive oil
1 lemon
3 large or 6 small garlic cloves, minced
1 shallot, diced
1 heaping tablespoon capers
2 tablespoons dried oregano
1 tablespoon dried basil

Preheat the oven to 350 degrees F.

Trim the excess fat and gristle from the chicken. It's all right if the chicken pieces vary in size. If the breasts are thick, carefully slice them laterally, so that they end up about half as thick (about ¼ inch each). Spread out the chicken slices and pieces in a baking pan. Next, add the chicken broth, then drizzle the olive oil over the chicken. Cut the lemon and squeeze the juice over the chicken. Add the garlic, shallot, capers, oregano, and basil. Bake for 30 to 35 minutes. This is an easy-to-prepare and very flavorful dinner and can be served with Pan-Fried Veggies (page 111) and Flavorful Brown Rice (page 109).

—☓—

Quick Tip: Using a Natural Salt

It is important for many people to reduce their intake of salt (sodium chloride). Unfortunately, most salt is added to foods during their manufacture, long before they reach the dining table. In Paleolithic times people consumed far more potassium than sodium, but today people tend to consume much more sodium than potassium. The biggest step in reducing your salt intake is to avoid processed and prepackaged foods, convenience foods, and fast foods. Unprocessed foods—fish, fowl, and vegetables—generally provide more potassium than sodium.

Still, if you would like to use a little salt—just a little—with your meals, try Celtic Sea Salt or RealSalt. Both products are mined from ancient salt beds and contain trace amounts of many minerals. They are available at nearly all health and natural food stores. For more information, go to www.realsalt.com.

—☓—

Evan's Chicken Schnitzel (*Serves 2 to 3*)

This meal is similar to a chicken-fried steak. Instead of using wheat flour or bread crumbs, however, you should use Lotus Foods' Bhutanese Red Rice Flour, which you can order directly from www.lotusfoods.com. The rice flour is much lighter than wheat, browns nicely, and adds a wonderful, rich flavor.

> 1 to 1½ pounds chicken breasts, boneless and skinless
> 1 egg, beaten in a bowl
> ¼ cup Bhutanese Red Rice Flour (potato flour can be substituted)
> olive oil
> pat of butter (optional)

Trim the excess fat and gristle from the chicken. Slice it into thin pieces, running the length of each chicken breast so the pieces are no more than about ¼ inch thick. Dip each piece into the egg, then dredge it through the flour. When all of the chicken pieces are prepared (you can prepare very small pieces of chicken similarly to minimize waste), heat the olive oil (and butter, if you choose) in a nonstick skillet. Place the chicken in the skillet and cook about 2 minutes or less per side. Serve with rice and your choice of vegetables.

Saffron Chicken Stir-Fry (*Serves 2 to 3*)

> ¼ to ½ teaspoon ground saffron
> ¼ cup water
> 1 to 1½ pounds chicken breast meat, skinless and boneless
> olive oil
> pat of butter (optional)
> 6 cloves garlic, minced
> juice of 1 to 1½ lemons

To grind the saffron: rub the strands between your fingers into a small bowl. Adding a pinch of salt will help you grind the saffron into a powder. Add the water (room temperature or warm) to the bowl with the saffron. Set it aside.

Slice or cube the chicken, removing unwanted fat and gristle. Coat a nonstick wok with olive oil (and butter if you wish) over medium heat. Add the chicken and begin stir-frying. When the chicken turns white, add the garlic and saffron mixture and continue to stir-fry for a couple more minutes. Add the lemon juice and stir-fry for another 1 or 2 minutes. The saffron mixture and lemon juice will prevent the chicken from drying out. Serve with rice and vegetables.

Spaghetti Squash Toss (*Serves 1 to 2*)

This makes a nice dinner for one or two people, plus leftovers that can be reheated in the microwave for lunch the next day.

> 1 medium-size spaghetti squash (2 to 2½ pounds)
> 1 boneless, skinless chicken breast or 10 to 20 shrimp and scallops
> olive oil
> 4 to 6 garlic cloves, minced
> 1 teaspoon basil
> 1 teaspoon oregano
> 2 to 3 ounces fresh baby spinach leaves
> juice of 1 to 2 lemons
> juice of 1 lime
> juice of ½ orange
> RealSalt (or Celtic Sea Salt) and black pepper

Bake the spaghetti squash for 1 hour or so, at 350 to 375 degrees F, until the skin is soft to the touch. (Use a pot holder or fork to touch it.) Remove the squash from the oven, cut it in half lengthwise, and use a spoon to scoop out the seeds. Run a fork along the fruit so that you create spaghettilike strands. While the squash is baking, stir-fry the chicken or shrimp and scallops in olive oil, along with the garlic, basil, and oregano in a skillet over medium heat. Add the spinach and continue to stir-fry. Add the lemon, lime, and orange juices when the chicken or seafood is almost cooked. Serve it on top of the spaghetti squash. Add salt and black pepper. The stir-frying should take no more than 5 to 10 minutes, so you can time it for when the squash will be ready.

—⚬—

Quick Tip: Quality Chicken Broths

When using packaged chicken broth in a recipe, quality makes a big difference. Health Valley and Pacific organic free-range chicken broths are simple and tasty, without thickeners, monosodium glutamate, and excessive amounts of salt. Both brands are available at natural foods grocery stores. Trader Joe's broths are made by Pacific.

—ɱ—

Baked Turkey Breast Provençal (*Serves 4*)

1 turkey breast, on bone or boneless (2½ to 3 pounds)
2 tablespoons olive oil, plus more as needed
herbes de Provence
rubbed or finely ground dried sage
chicken broth
2 bay leaves
juice of 1 lemon
water

Preheat the oven to 350 degrees F.

Place the turkey breast in a deep roasting pan, and use your hands to separate but not completely detach the skin from the top of the turkey. Rub a little olive oil on the turkey to keep it from burning or drying out. Sprinkle on the herbes de Provence and sage, then place the skin over the spices. You may add a little more olive oil and spices to the skin if you wish. Add about ½ inch high-quality chicken broth (such as Health Valley or Pacific organic free-range chicken broth) to the bottom of the pot. Add a little more of the spices, plus the bay leaves, 2 tablespoons of olive oil, and lemon juice. Bake it uncovered for 30 to 40 minutes per pound, approximately 90 minutes to 2 hours total. Add water every 30 minutes or so to maintain the level of the broth, which will become your au jus. During the final 30 minutes, cover the pot. Save the leftover turkey and au jus for other meals or recipes, such as Turkey Rice Soup (page 116).

Saffron Seafood Soup (*Serves 4*)

1 small onion, finely diced
1 leek, very thinly sliced (white part only)
1 carrot, thinly sliced
2 teaspoons butter

½ cup dry vermouth or dry white wine
3 to 4 cups fish stock
1 cup short-grain brown rice, already cooked
pinch ground saffron
½ teaspoon dried dill or Deliciously Dill seasoning
½ to 1 cup heavy cream
4 ounces salmon fillet, cut into small pieces
6 to 8 large shrimp, cut into small pieces
1 to 2 oysters, shucked and rinsed
½ teaspoon RealSalt or Celtic Sea Salt

Sauté the onion, leek, and carrot in butter in a large pan over medium heat. When they soften (3 to 5 minutes), add the vermouth, fish stock, rice, and saffron. Bring this to a boil, then add the dill, reduce the heat, and let simmer for 10 to 15 minutes. (If you prefer to have a thick rather than chunky soup, allow it to cool slightly and pureé it in a blender until smooth, then continue simmering.) Stir the cream into the simmering soup, then add the salmon, shrimp, oysters, and RealSalt or Celtic Sea Salt. Simmer for another 3 to 5 minutes until the fish is cooked and tender.

Curry Dishes

Curries are rich in powerful anti-inflammatory spices, such as turmeric, coriander, and cumin. Over the last few years, I have found myself cooking many Thai and Indian curry dishes at home because they are relatively easy. For Thai curries, I simplify things by using Thai Kitchen's red and green curry pastes as the spice base, although I will often add additional curry or cayenne spices. You can buy Thai Kitchen pastes at many supermarkets and online at www.worldpantry.com. Alternatively, you can buy Blue Elephant green, red, and yellow curry pastes, although they do contain a small amount of soybean oil. The Blue Elephant curry pastes were developed by the Blue Elephant restaurants in London, Paris, Copenhagen, and other cities, and you can find the pastes at Cost Plus World Market stores in the United States.

Shrimp in Thai Green Curry (*Serves 4*)

1 tablespoon macadamia nut oil or coconut oil
2 to 3 cloves garlic, sliced thinly

10 to 15 baby asparagus spears, fresh or frozen and defrosted
1 12-ounce can coconut milk (not lite)
1 tablespoon Thai Kitchen Green Curry Paste
½ teaspoon turmeric
½ teaspoon red pepper flakes
1 pound shrimp, fresh or frozen and defrosted
½ teaspoon Thai Kitchen fish sauce (optional)
¼ cup fresh basil leaves

Heat the oil in a deep skillet over high heat and, when hot, sauté the garlic and asparagus until a little soft. Slowly pour the coconut milk into the skillet, then add the Thai Kitchen Green Curry Paste, turmeric, and red pepper flakes. Using a spatula, thoroughly mix the paste into the coconut milk, while bringing it to a light boil. Add the shrimp and stir it just a little so that all of the shrimp are covered by the coconut milk. Add the fish sauce, if using. Cover the skillet (use aluminum foil if you don't have a lid), turn the heat down to medium, and cook for 10 minutes, stirring occasionally. Add the basil leaves and cook for about 1 minute more. Serve with steamed cauliflower and brown or purple Forbidden Rice.

Chicken in Thai Red Curry (*Serves 4*)

1 tablespoon macadamia nut oil or coconut oil
2 to 3 cloves garlic, sliced thinly
½ cup diced eggplant (about ¼ inch cubes)
1 12-ounce can coconut milk (not lite)
1 tablespoon Thai Kitchen Red Curry Paste
½ teaspoon turmeric
½ teaspoon red pepper flakes
1 to 1 ½ pounds boneless, skinless chicken breast, cut into cubes or
    slices
½ teaspoon Thai Kitchen fish sauce (optional)
¼ cup fresh basil leaves

Heat the macadamia nut oil in a deep skillet over high heat and, when hot, sauté the garlic and eggplant until they're soft. Slowly pour the coconut milk into the skillet, then add the Thai Kitchen Red Curry Paste, turmeric, and red pepper flakes. Using a spatula, thoroughly mix the paste into the coconut milk, while bringing it to a light boil. Add the chicken, and stir it just a little so that all of it is covered by the coconut milk. Add the fish sauce, if using. Cover the skillet (use aluminum foil if you don't have a lid), turn the heat down to medium, and cook for 15 minutes, stirring occasionally. Add the basil leaves and cook for about 1 minute more. Serve with steamed cauliflower and brown or purple Forbidden Rice.

Curried Chicken Salad (*Serves 4+*)

Chicken salad doesn't have to be boring. This recipe uses Indian (rather than Thai) ingredients, and it's one of my favorite recipes. It will forever change your thinking about ho-hum chicken salad.

> 2½ to 3 cups (1 to 1.5 pounds) chicken, cooked, cooled, and diced
> 1 cup diced celery
> ½ cup organic raisins
> ½ cup raw almond slices
> 1 to 2 teaspoons curry powder
> ¼ to ½ teaspoon ground cayenne pepper (depending on how hot you want it)
> 1 to 2 teaspoons apple cider vinegar
> ½ to 1 cup high-quality canola or olive-oil mayonnaise (e.g., Spectrum Naturals)

Combine the chicken, celery, raisins, and almond slices in a large bowl and mix together with a large spoon. Add the curry powder and cayenne pepper and mix the ingredients together again. Now drizzle on the vinegar and add the mayonnaise, starting with about ½ cup and adding more mayonnaise to suit your personal preference for creaminess. Allow the ingredients to sit in the refrigerator for 1 to 2 hours before serving, to enable flavors to integrate. You can substitute diced turkey for the chicken.

Lamb Curry (*Serves 4*)

> macadamia nut oil or avocado oil
> 1 to 1¼ pounds lamb cubes or ground lamb
> 1 medium to large red onion, chopped
> 2 to 4 cloves garlic, chopped
> 1 tablespoon diced fresh ginger

1 pat butter, plus more if needed
1 tablespoon curry powder spice blend
½ teaspoon cumin
½ teaspoon turmeric
¼ teaspoon cayenne pepper
1 to 2 cups baby spinach leaves (optional)
1 cup chicken broth
1 cup unsweetened yogurt
Celtic Sea Salt or RealSalt

Heat about 1 tablespoon of either avocado oil or macadamia nut oil in a 2- or 3-quart pan over high heat, then add the lamb. (If you use ground lamb, break it into small chunklike pieces.) When it's cooked or mostly cooked, drain off the fat and transfer the lamb to a bowl. Next, prepare an Indian "roux" (pronounced *roo*) by sautéing the onion, garlic, and ginger in a pat of butter and a little oil until they're soft. Add more butter and oil as needed to keep the ingredients from burning. When the onion, garlic, and ginger soften, turn down the heat to medium. Add the lamb, followed by the curry powder, cumin, turmeric, and cayenne pepper, stirring all of the ingredients together. (If using, add the baby spinach leaves at this point.) Add the chicken broth and stir. Turn the heat down a little more, add the yogurt, and stir everything together. Add salt.

Note: You can substitute chicken and shrimp in this recipe, but skip the extra cumin.

Curry Powder

In Thailand, India, and other nations of southern and southeastern Asia, families blend spices to make curry powder. In the United States, most grocers sell a generic curry powder that works reasonably well, although I prefer to add some spices to this mix. A little extra cumin adds an earthiness to the flavor without adding heat. Turmeric contains the anti-inflammatory curcumin. If you would like to make your own curry powder, start with this recipe.

¼ cup or so ground cumin
¼ cup ground coriander
⅛ cup ground cardamom
1 tablespoon ground black peppercorns

1 tablespoon ground turmeric
1 teaspoon ground cloves
1 teaspoon ground fennel seeds (optional)

Blend all of the ingredients in a bowl. Store the powder in a container with a tightly fitted lid. It will keep up to 1 year refrigerated. Use as needed for recipes and as a seasoning.

—⟋⟍—

A Source for Culinary Spices

One of the best sources of fresh bulk spices is the Spice House, which operates five retail stores in the Chicago area and Milwaukee. Most of the Spice House's herbs and spices are sold in bulk, although a few are bottled for the convenience of customers. The Spice House has several curry blends from mild (called "sweet curry," although it has no sugar) to several varieties of hot curries. The stores sell hundreds of other spices, which you can order and have shipped to you. For more information, visit www.thespicehouse.com or call (847) 328-3711.

—⟋⟍—

Side Dishes

Spinach and Leek Sauté (*Serves 1 to 2*)

1 6-ounce bag fresh spinach
1 leek, white part only
2 pats butter
water
1 tablespoon pine nuts
garlic powder

Pinch the stems from the spinach leaves and place the leaves in a large colander. Slice the leek into pieces just over the thickness of a quarter. In a 10-inch nonstick skillet, over medium heat, sauté the leek with a pat of butter until the leek starts to caramelize. Meanwhile, boil a pot of water and pour it over the spinach in the colander. This will gently wilt and compress the spinach. Allow the spinach to cool a little, then press out the excess water. When the leek has caramelized, add the other pat of butter and then the spinach; you may need to use a fork to separate the clumps of spinach. Sauté the vegetables and add the pine nuts and garlic powder.

This is a modest vegetable side dish for two people that goes well with Baked Salmon (page 96). Quantities can easily be doubled.

Flavorful Brown Rice (*Serves 2*)

Short-grain brown rice has a wonderful flavor, and at the table you can add a small amount of RealSalt or Celtic Sea Salt and butter to taste.

> 1 cup short-grain brown rice
> 1 cup chicken broth (or water)
> 1 cup water

Rinse the rice in a strainer, then put it in a 2-quart pan. Add the broth and water (or simply water if you're not using broth). Use very high heat and boil for 5 minutes, then turn the heat down to simmer. The rice should cook fully in about 40 minutes; you may have to adjust the heat above a simmer to accomplish this.

As a variation, consider sautéing some finely diced shallots, garlic, and onions in as little olive oil as possible, then mixing them into the rice before you start to cook it.

—⚉—

Quick Tip: Nice Rice

Tired of the same old rice? White rice is pretty bland (and nothing more than pure carbohydrate), but brown rice can get a little boring after a while too. Lotus Foods (www.lotusfoods.com) markets a selection of rich-tasting rices from Asia that are unlike any other type of rice. The company's Bhutanese Red Rice is a tasty red rice, and Forbidden Rice is a flavorful purple-colored rice. Both types cook faster than brown rice and require less broth (or water), so be careful to follow label directions. Both rices, and others, are also available as flours.

—⚉—

Purple Rice (*Serves 4*)

> 1 cup purple rice (such as Lotus Foods' Forbidden Rice,
>   www.lotusfoods.com)
> 1 cup organic/free-range chicken broth
> ¾ cup water

Rinse the rice in a strainer and transfer it to a 1- or 2-quart pan. Add the chicken broth and water. Bring this to a boil over high heat, about 5 minutes. Cover and reduce the heat to a simmer for about 30 minutes, until the rice is fully cooked.

Wild Rice (*Serves 4*)

> 1 cup wild rice
> 1 cup high-quality chicken or vegetable broth
> 2 cups water
> 2 stalks celery, diced
> 4 ounces water chestnuts, diced
> 2 to 3 tablespoons organic raisins

Wild rice is actually a grass, not a rice. It has a full-bodied flavor.

Rinse the rice in a strainer and transfer it to a 1- or 2-quart pan. Add the broth and water. Bring this to a boil over high heat (about 5 minutes), then cover and reduce the heat to a simmer. After 20 minutes, add the celery, water chestnuts, and raisins to the rice and stir. The rice should be fully cooked in 40 to 50 minutes. Fluff it with a fork and drain off any excess water. The rice should be al dente; do not overcook it.

Cauliflower and Broccoli (*Serves 2*)

> ½ head cauliflower
> ½ bunch broccoli
> ½ stick (⅛ pound) butter
> 2 to 3 tablespoons pine nuts, sliced almonds, or pecan or
>   hazelnut pieces

Cut the cauliflower and broccoli into florets about ½ to 1 inch in diameter. Steam them in a pot for 10 minutes over high heat. While doing this, melt the butter in a pan, then add the nuts of your choice. Transfer the cauliflower and broccoli to a bowl, then pour the butter/nut mixture over them and toss. Serve the dish immediately.

Pan-Fried Veggies (*Serves 2*)

¼ cup olive oil
1 pat unsalted butter (optional)
1 or 2 small zucchini
1 cup frozen corn kernels
1 large garlic clove, diced
1 scallion, diced
¼ teaspoon garlic powder
½ teaspoon dried oregano
½ teaspoon dried basil
¼ cup pine nuts
1 tablespoon golden raisins

Add the olive oil and butter to a 10-inch skillet or wok. Cut the tops and bottoms off the zucchini, quarter them lengthwise, and dice so that the pieces are roughly the size of dimes, but a little thicker. Put the zucchini into the pan, along with the corn and diced garlic, scallion, garlic powder, oregano, and basil. With a spatula, mix everything around as you start to heat the vegetables at a medium setting. Cover the pan (loosely with a piece of aluminum foil if you don't have a lid). Stir every couple of minutes. After about 5 minutes, add the pine nuts. Cook until the zucchini softens and the corn starts to turn brown and caramelize. After a few minutes more, add the raisins and let cook for 10 to 15 minutes more, stirring occasionally. This is an easy side dish and goes great with Wonderful Baked Chicken Breasts (page 100).

—⁓—

Quick Tip: The Secret of Tomato-Free Ratatouille

Traditional ratatouille consists of sautéed vegetables, including tomatoes. The following recipe avoids tomatoes, a nightshade plant that can aggravate arthritic symptoms in some people. Instead, it uses tomatillos (*Physalis ixocarpa*), also known as Mexican green tomatoes. Tomatillos, which can be bought fresh or canned at supermarkets, are also members of the nightshade family, but they are more closely related to the Cape gooseberry than to tomatoes. If you are very sensitive to nightshades, substitute extra zucchini for the eggplant (another nightshade), and test whether you are sensitive to tomatillos. All of these vegetables cook down, so use a large, covered, nonstick, woklike pan. The amounts below can easily be doubled, allowing the ratatouille to be used as a vegetable side dish and with breakfasts as well. See the Omelet with Tomato-Free Ratatouille Filling recipe (page 117). *Note*: If you react to all nightshade plants, this is not a recipe you should try.

—⁓—

Tomato-Free Ratatouille (*Serves 2 to 3*)

¼ to ½ cup olive oil
2 small or 1 large eggplant, diced
1 large bell pepper, or the equivalent from several colored
    varieties, diced
2 zucchinis, each originally about 10 inches long, diced
1 medium red or sweet onion, diced
1 to 2 teaspoons thyme
1 to 2 teaspoons basil
1 bay leaf
4 garlic cloves, finely minced
3 to 4 ripe tomatillos (should have yellow-green lime color),
    diced
Celtic Sea Salt, RealSalt, or sea salt

Pour about ¼ cup of olive oil into a pan over medium heat. When the olive oil is warm, add the eggplant, stirring occasionally. The eggplant will soak up the olive oil, but keep the pan covered to retain moisture. Add the bell pepper, zucchinis, and onion. After a few minutes, add the thyme, basil, bay leaf, garlic, and tomatillos. Stir occasionally to keep the vegetables from burning, and keep the pan covered when you are not stirring. Add a little more olive oil if necessary. Turn the heat down and allow everything to simmer for about 40 minutes or until all of the vegetables are very soft. Add Celtic Sea Salt, RealSalt, or regular sea salt. Dispose of the bay leaf before serving.

Mashed Cauliflower with Turmeric (*Serves 3 to 4*)

1 to 1½ pounds cauliflower
1 teaspoon curry powder blend
¼ teaspoon ground turmeric
Celtic Sea Salt, Real Salt, or sea salt
freshly ground black pepper

Cut the cauliflower into florets and steam them until soft, 15 to 20 minutes. Remove the florets from the steamer, place them in a bowl, and mash the cauliflower as you would potatoes. Sprinkle it with the curry powder and turmeric and mix well with a fork. Add salt and pepper. *Tip:* You can use some of the cauliflower leftovers in an omelet or scrambled eggs.

Green Bean and Mushroom Stir-Fry (*Serves 2*)

1 pat butter
2 tablespoons olive oil
2 handfuls fresh or frozen green beans, ideally French cut
4 to 5 fresh mushrooms, sliced
garlic powder
⅛ cup sliced almonds

Heat the butter and olive oil in a nonstick skillet or a wok over medium heat. Add the green beans and cook until they start to get soft. Add the mushroom slices and garlic powder. When the green beans and mushrooms are almost cooked, add the sliced almonds.

Mushroom and Spinach Sauté (*Serves 1*)

olive oil
6 to 10 small mushrooms, sliced
3 small scallions, diced
3 ounces (about ½ bag) fresh spinach
garlic powder

Coat a nonstick skillet with olive oil, add the mushrooms and scallions, and sauté over medium heat. Meanwhile, pinch the stems from the spinach leaves (or leave them on, if you prefer). When the mushrooms and scallions soften, add the spinach, then add the garlic powder. Stir to thoroughly mix the vegetables together. For variety, use a different type of mushroom, such as shiitake or chanterelle.

Tangy Butternut Squash (*Serves 2*)

> 1 to 2 butternut squashes
> 1 teaspoon walnut, hazelnut, or olive oil, plus more as needed
> ½ to 1 teaspoon dried thyme, plus more as needed
> ½ teaspoon balsamic vinegar, plus more as needed

Preheat the oven to 350 degrees F.

Cut off the tip of the squash stem, then cut the squash in half lengthwise. Remove the seeds with a spoon (a serrated grapefruit spoon works well). Lightly coat the inside of the squash with olive oil to minimize burning. Place the squash cut side down (skin side up) in a baking pan, and bake for approximately 1 hour. The squash is cooked when the skin is tender to the touch. (Use a fork or a spoon to touch, not your hand.) Remove the squash from the oven, scrape the pulp with a spoon, and place the pulp in a bowl. Add about ½ teaspoon of thyme per squash, plus about 1 teaspoon of walnut or other oil and about ½ teaspoon of balsamic vinegar. Mix everything together with a fork, adding additional thyme, oil, or vinegar to suit your taste.

Lunch Meals

Turkey Tacos (*Serves 4*)

> taco seasoning
> about 1 teaspoon olive oil
> 1 pound ground turkey
> ¾ cup water
> low-carb whole-wheat tortillas, sour cream, guacamole,
>   diced scallions, and tomatoes (optional)

Use either my seasoning blend (recipe below) or McCormick's Taco Seasoning Mix. Heat the olive oil in a large skillet over medium-high heat. Break up the ground turkey into small chunky pieces and cook it thoroughly, about 5 minutes. Drain off the fat and reduce the heat. Add the taco seasoning mix and water, then stir to blend the spices with the meat. Reduce the heat to a simmer. To serve, roll the mixture in a low-carb whole-wheat tortilla. Alternatively, transfer some of the cooked turkey taco to a plate, add a dollop of sour cream or guacamole, and sprinkle on some diced scallions and tomatoes.

Jack's Taco Seasoning Blend

Most commercial taco seasoning blends have undesirable ingredients, such as too much salt or wheat (added as a thickener), although McCormick's Taco Seasoning Mix is probably the "nutritionally clean-est" of them. It's easy, however, to make your own. In a bowl, mix together the following ingredients, but the first time you make it, add the cayenne pepper slowly to determine your preferred level of heat.

 1 teaspoon ground cumin
 1 teaspoon ground oregano
 ½ teaspoon onion powder
 ½ teaspoon garlic powder
 ½ teaspoon paprika
 ¼ to ½ teaspoon cayenne pepper (ground)
 ¼ to ½ teaspoon cayenne pepper flakes

Wonderful Whatever Salad (*Serves 1*)

 any green leafy lettuce (not iceberg) or spinach
 cucumber
 scallion, diced
 tomato or bell peppers
 sliced almonds
 artichoke hearts (packed in water, not oil)
 hemp nut seeds
 cooked chicken or turkey, diced, or pieces of poached salmon

No amounts are given because they are purely at your discretion. Prepare the ingredients in the desired amounts and toss. Avoid dressings with soybean oil or hydrogenated vegetable oil. Two recommended salad dressings are Stonewall Kitchen Roasted Garlic Vinaigrette (www.stonewall kitchen.com) and Zeus Greek Salad Dressing (www.zeusfoods.com).

Quick Chicken or Turkey Rice Soup (*Serves 2*)

This soup is a creative and tasty use of leftover chicken or turkey, regardless of how it was originally prepared.

> 2 cups chicken broth
> 2 ounces cooked chicken or turkey, diced
> ½ cup cooked short-grain brown rice
> 1 scallion, diced
> ⅓ cup diced mushrooms
> garlic powder
> Celtic Sea Salt or RealSalt
> black pepper

Pour the chicken broth in a pan and begin to heat it. Add the chicken or turkey to the broth along with the rice, scallions, and mushrooms. Stir occasionally and bring it to a light boil. Serve, adding the garlic powder, salt, and pepper at the table.

Breakfasts

Breakfast Scramble (*Serves 1–2*)

> olive oil or butter
> 1 scallion, diced, per person
> spinach (either fresh with stems removed or defrosted)
> 2 tablespoons cooked brown rice
> 1 to 2 tablespoons leftover chicken or turkey, diced
> 2 eggs, beaten, per person

Heat the olive oil or butter in a skillet and sauté the scallions over medium heat until they soften. Add the spinach, brown rice, and chicken or turkey. When the spinach is wilted, pour in the eggs and mix everything thoroughly with a spatula. Serve it when the eggs are cooked. Serve fresh fruit as a side dish.

Omelet with Tomato-Free Ratatouille Filling (*Serves 1*)

>1 pat of butter or a little olive oil
>2 to 3 eggs
>2 tablespoons Tomato-Free Ratatouille (page 112)

Heat a pat of butter or a little olive oil in a skillet. Beat the eggs, pour them into the pan, and begin cooking them as a plain omelet. Meanwhile, heat the Tomato-Free Ratatouille on a small plate in a microwave. After you flip the omelet, spoon the ratatouille onto one side, then fold over the omelet. Serve with fresh fruit, such as berries or apple slices.

Breakfast Mini Chicken Patties (*Serves 2 to 3*)

>1 pound ground chicken (or turkey)
>4 cloves garlic, minced
>4 pitted olives, finely chopped
>1 tablespoon oregano
>1 tablespoon basil

Preheat the oven to 350 degrees F.

Put the ground chicken in a bowl. (Many natural foods grocers sell ground chicken, frozen, in 1-pound packages.) Add the garlic, olives, oregano, and basil. Mix everything thoroughly with your hands (wear disposable gloves) and form patties about ¼ inch thick and about 1½ to 2 inches in diameter. One pound of ground chicken should yield about a dozen patties, although you can make them smaller. Place the patties in a baking dish and bake for 20 minutes. When they're done, soak up the extra fat with paper towels.

Tip: Follow the same recipe to make chickenburgers comparable to the size of a hamburger. Use different types of pitted olives (such as green or Kalamata) to vary the flavor. You also can substitute ground turkey for ground chicken.

Breakfast Muesli (*Serves 1*)

This breakfast takes about 5 minutes to prepare the night before and is ready in about 2 minutes in the morning. Mix ⅓ cup of muesli with about ½ cup of coconut milk, water, or milk (if you are not allergic to dairy) in a small bowl. Cover the bowl, and leave it in the refrigerator overnight. Meanwhile, defrost a total of 2 to 3 tablespoons of raspberries and blueberries overnight, or be sure to have some fresh fruit on hand for the morning, such as berries, an apple, or a banana. In the morning add the fruit (dice the apple or banana) and mix it into the muesli. Add a little cinnamon or a very small amount of nutmeg for flavoring. Eat it as a side dish with a few reheated Breakfast Mini Chicken Patties (above).

Baked Sweet Potatoes or Yams (*Serves 1 to 2*)

> 1 to 2 sweet potatoes or yams
> butter
> 1 tablespoon finely chopped fresh chives or scallions
> salt

Preheat the oven to 375 degrees F.

Place the sweet potatoes on aluminum foil and bake for 1 to 1½ hours, depending on their size. Cut them in half and serve as you would a baked potato, with butter and chives or scallions. Add salt.

Sample Two-Week-Long Meal Plan

This meal plan is *not* intended to be a rigid you-must-follow-or-else dietary plan. Rather, it is just what the name says—a sample of what you might choose to cook, reuse as creative leftovers, or order in a restaurant. The key is following, at every meal, the dietary principles discussed in chapter 6. An asterisk indicates that the recipe is included in this chapter.

Day 1

Breakfast	Breakfast Scramble,* fresh fruit, and a wheat-free waffle with almond butter
Lunch	In a restaurant, order a grilled chicken breast, minus the bun, and a side of vegetables instead of fries; sparkling water to drink
Dinner	Baked Salmon,* Spinach and Leek Sauté,* and rice

Day 2

Breakfast   Breakfast Mini Chicken Patties,* fresh fruit, and sliced gluten-free bread, toasted and spread with almond butter

Lunch   Wonderful Whatever Salad,* with leftover pieces of salmon from last evening's dinner

Dinner   Baked Turkey Breast Provençal,* Mushroom and Spinach Sauté,* and rice or baked squash

Day 3

Breakfast   Leftover Breakfast Mini Chicken Patties,* and Breakfast Muesli* with fruit

Lunch   Reheated turkey with au jus, Spinach and Leek Sauté,* and rice

Dinner   Pumpkin Seed–Crusted Halibut,* Green Bean and Mushroom Stir-Fry,* and Forbidden Rice and spinach salad on the side

Day 4

Breakfast   Omelette with Tomato-Free Ratatouille Filling, and fresh fruit

Lunch   Quick Chicken or Turkey Rice Soup,* and a side salad with butter lettuce

Dinner   In a restaurant, order baked or broiled fish with vegetables and a small green salad

Day 5

Breakfast   Omelette with baby shrimp and sautéed scallions and spinach

Lunch   Salmon or halibut fish patty (see "Specialty Foods" in the appendix at www.inflammationsyndrome.com), Green Bean and Mushroom Stir-Fry,* rice, and a small green salad

Dinner   Pan-Fried Swordfish,* steamed cauliflower and broccoli, and rice

Day 6

Breakfast   Breakfast Scramble* with diced turkey

Lunch   Wonderful Whatever Salad* with leftover diced turkey

Dinner   Wonderful Baked Chicken Breasts,* Green Bean and Mushroom Stir-Fry,* rice, and a small green salad

Day 7

Breakfast   Breakfast Scramble* using diced chicken and small amounts of the Green Bean and Mushroom Stir-Fry* and rice from last evening's dinner

Lunch   Tuna salad with salad greens

Dinner   Baked Shrimp and Scallops,* or your choice of rice or vegetable, stir-fried

Day 8

Breakfast   Steel-cut oatmeal with cinnamon powder and blueberries

Lunch   Chicken Caesar salad (sans croutons)

Dinner   Turkey Tacos*

Day 9

Breakfast   Turkey Taco and egg burrito in a low-carb whole-wheat tortilla

Lunch   Curried Chicken Salad*

Dinner   Halibut grilled with butter and olive oil

Day 10

Breakfast   Roast beef or turkey slices with sliced cheese, and an apple on the side

Lunch   Marinated shrimp and cucumber salad

Dinner   Poached Salmon in Garlic-Infused Olive Oil*

Day 11

Breakfast   Scrambled eggs with leftover Turkey Tacos

Lunch   Chicken breast and steamed vegetables

Dinner   Sautéed scallops with lemon butter and oregano sauce

Day 12

Breakfast   Omelet stuffed with chives and organic cream cheese

Lunch   Hamburger (no bun), with steamed cauliflower

Dinner   Shrimp in Thai Green Curry*

Day 13

Breakfast   Omelet with leftover Shrimp in Thai Green Curry

Lunch   Quick Chicken Rice Soup

Dinner   Roasted Salmon*

Day 14
Breakfast   Scrambled egg with cooked brown rice and Romano cheese
Lunch   Salmon burgers
Dinner   Lamb Curry*

Beverages, Snacks, and Desserts

Often people stray from a diet when choosing beverages, snacks, and desserts. Here are some suggestions to keep things simple and to help you stay on the AI Diet Plan.

Some research has found that people consuming sugar-free diet soft drinks gain as much weight as those who drink the same amounts of sugary drinks. Diet soft drinks may delude us into thinking we can eat other high-calorie foods, such as pizzas, but the final calorie count between food and beverages ends up about equal. Meanwhile, other research suggests that high-fructose corn syrup, the sweetener now found in most soft drinks, affects the appetite centers of the brain and triggers increased consumption. Yet other research indicates that the higher fructose component of high-fructose corn syrup increases fat production in the body.

For cold beverages, I recommend sparkling mineral or still waters with a wedge of lemon, lime, or orange for flavoring. Mineral waters are rich in calcium, magnesium, and bicarbonate. Trader Joe's and many supermarkets sell a variety of sparking mineral waters, including Perrier, San Pellegrino, Gerolsteiner, and others. Still (nonbubbly) mineral waters are more difficult to find in the United States, compared with Europe, but the Cost Plus World Market chain of stores sells several brands. The best-tasting still mineral waters are Hildon, Ty Nant, and Voss. Do note that most of the still waters sold in plastic bottles are not mineral waters.

Another option consists of iced green tea and various herbal teas, which can be brewed in a pitcher on a countertop or as sun teas. I recommend a specific type of green tea sold by Miroku. (See the appendix at www.inflammationsyndrome.com.) Read the labels of tea blends carefully because some may contain added sweeteners, calories you just don't need.

Yet another option consists of coconut water, sold in 11-ounce packets at many health food markets. The tastiest brand is ZICO, but O.N.E. and Harvest Bay are also very good. (Again, see the appendix at www.inflammationsyndrome.com.) Coconut water contains no fat (unlike coconut oil or coconut milk) and is rich in potassium, which may have anti-inflammatory benefits. Food sources of potassium are safe, whereas high doses of potassium supplements may negatively affect heart rhythm.

Snack foods often derail the best intentions. I recommend making your own trail mix with a blend of unsalted, roasted, or raw nuts and seeds. You can include any combination of almonds, macadamias, pistachios, pumpkin seeds, sunflower seeds, and organic raisins. Mix them together in a large bowl and then transfer them to small plastic bags that you can keep in the office or in your car. Another option is based on a Morrocan appetizer: one or two dried figs with a half-dozen raw almonds.

Fresh Ginger Tea (*Serves 1*)

Ginger is a potent anti-inflammatory, and I prefer making this simple ginger tea to taking capsules.

    fresh ginger root
    1 mug water
    1 cinnamon stick (optional)

Use a vegetable peeler to remove the skin of a small piece of ginger root. Then use the peeler to cut 10 to 20 slices of the ginger root (each slice should be about 1 inch or so long). Place the ginger in a mug. Heat some water in a pot, then pour it into the mug and allow the ginger to steep for a few minutes; or pour water into the mug and microwave it until hot. Allow the tea to cool down a little before drinking it. You can also add a cinnamon stick. When the tea is gone, you can chew on some of the ginger pieces.

PART III

The AI
Supplement Plan

CHAPTER 8

Good Fats That Rev Up Your Body's Natural Anti-Inflammatories

Anita: Fish Oil for Lower Blood Pressure

Anita was a widowed single mother who looked much older than her thirty-six years. The pressures of working and mothering three young children forced her to stop making home-cooked meals in favor of giving her kids burgers, fries, pizzas, and quick-energy foods such as candy bars and soft drinks. At the end of each day she collapsed into bed, exhausted and drained.

Over two years, Anita had gained thirty pounds and now experienced frequent headaches and suffered joint pain in her hips, shoulders, and hands. Her medical doctor prescribed ibuprofen, and a rheumatologist told her she had some (but not all) of the signs of lupus erythematosus. She was developing stomach pain from the ibuprofen, and medications for the lupuslike symptoms caused double vision. Anita's blood pressure had risen to 190/100 and her blood sugar was more than 240, clearly in the diabetic range. These clinical findings led to additional prescriptions for hypertensive and glucose-lowering medications.

A friend recommended that Anita consult with Judy A. Heill, N.D., a naturopathic physician in Tucson, Arizona. After a workup Heill asked

Anita to follow a simple, wholesome diet similar to the AI Diet Plan. Anita began eating more fish, chicken, turkey, and vegetables, while avoiding processed foods, soft drinks, coffee, and dairy products. Heill also asked her to take several anti-inflammatory supplements, including fish oil capsules (1,000 mg twice daily), as well as ginger, turmeric, and bromelain.

Anita's response was dramatic. After three weeks she had lost ten pounds and her glucose had normalized, enabling her to stop taking the glucose-lowering medications. Her pain, swelling, and stiffness decreased considerably, and her energy levels began to increase. At a six-week follow-up visit Anita had lost a total of eighteen pounds, and her blood pressure was normal, so she was able to stop taking the hypertensive medications. In addition, her joint pain was almost entirely gone, flaring up only when she went off her diet of simple, wholesome foods. Anita no longer had a need to take cortisone drugs for her lupuslike symptoms. Her headaches were gone, her energy levels were better, and she actually looked younger.

Omega-3 Fish Oils

You read in chapter 3 that the omega-3 fatty acids form the building blocks of many of the body's natural, innate analgesic substances. Fish oil supplements, which are produced from salmon and other varieties of coldwater fish, are rich in eicosapentaenoic acid (EPA) and docosahexaenoic acid (DHA). Both fatty acids are essential for health and play roles in the body's defenses against inflammation.

If the research on omega-3 fatty acids were seen in political terms, it would amount to a landslide victory. More than 8,000 scientific and medical articles have been published on the omega-3s, and medical journals currently publish approximately 800 news articles on the omega-3s each year. The omega-3s protect against heart diseases, cancer, Alzheimer's, mood disorders, arthritis, eye diseases, and numerous other health problems. It's no wonder they frequently garner bold newspaper headlines.

The advantage of taking fish oil capsules is simple: your body does *not* have to convert alpha-linolenic acid to EPA and DHA. As a result, supplements leapfrog several troublesome biochemical steps and bottlenecks. Your body quickly converts EPA and DHA to a variety of very potent anti-inflammatory compounds, including prostaglandin E_3, leukotriene B_5, resolvins, and protectins. These compounds counteract and suppress a variety of pro-inflammatory substances, including prostaglandin E_2, thromboxane B_2, interleukin-6, and C-reactive protein.

Fish Oils Protect against Heart Disease

One key discovery that led up to the concept of the inflammation syndrome was the medical recognition that chronic, low-grade inflammation (rather than cholesterol) causes coronary heart disease. It shouldn't be surprising, then, that eating fish or taking fish oil capsules is a phenomenal way to reduce inflammation and the risk of developing heart diseases. The cardiovascular benefits of omega-3 fish oils derive directly from the anti-inflammatory effects of EPA and DHA.

The modern story of omega-3 fish oils began in 1973, when Danish researchers investigated why traditional Eskimos who followed a high-fat diet were less likely to develop heart disease, compared with Eskimos who had a Western diet with meat and dairy foods. The researchers determined that the traditional Eskimo diet included large amounts of omega-3 fatty acids. Another study along these lines, published in 2001, found that Canadian Eskimos who had a traditional diet, including fish and marine mammals, had half the incidence of cardiovascular-related deaths, compared with other Canadians.

- *Coronary heart disease.* An analysis of studies, reported in the June 2008 *American Journal of Clinical Nutrition*, concluded that a modest consumption of fish (one or two servings weekly) reduced the risk of deaths from coronary heart disease by more than one-third. Meanwhile, a large European study found that omega-3 fish oil supplements led to significant reductions in cardiovascular-related deaths, heart attacks, and strokes.
- *Triglycerides.* High levels of these blood fats are a major risk factor for developing heart disease. Omega-3 fish oils are so effective at lowering triglycerides that the Food and Drug Administration has approved a "drug" version of omega-3s (called Lovaza) to reduce triglyceride levels. The drug costs $4 a day (for four capsules of Lovaza), compared with about 40¢ a day for over-the-counter fish oils that are just as good.
- *Coagulation.* The omega-3 fish oils have a mild blood-thinning effect, which reduces the risk of developing blood clots in arteries. Fish oil supplements (3 grams daily) can lower levels of fibrinogen and other clotting factors.
- *Blood pressure.* Omega-3 fish oils have a moderate blood pressure–lowering benefit, particularly in people who have both hypertension and high cholesterol levels.

- *Heart rate and rhythm.* The omega-3s have long been known to reduce the risk of erratic heartbeats called arrhythmias. In a study published in the *British Journal of Nutrition*, researchers gave fish oil supplements or placebos to sixty-five overweight and sedentary adults. Fish oils decreased the subjects' resting heart rates and also reduced abnormal variability in their heart rates. In other research, fish oil supplements decreased the risk of fatal arrhythmias by almost 30 percent.
- *Benefits during and after heart surgery.* Surgeons and anesthesiologists typically discourage patients from taking nutritional supplements. In a recent study, however, European researchers gave 8 grams of omega-3 fish oil capsules daily to coronary artery bypass patients. The fish oils led to decreases in the patients' "bad" very-low-density lipoprotein (VLDL) cholesterol and increases in their "good" high-density lipoprotein (HDL) cholesterol. Another benefit: the patients had low levels of troponin, a marker of surgery-related heart damage.

Fish Oils Protect against Osteoarthritis

Fish oil supplements may halt the breakdown of joint cartilage. Bruce Caterson, Ph.D., of Cardiff University, Wales, found that the omega-3 fatty acids inhibit the activity of aggrecanases, a family of enzymes that breaks down cartilage. In his experiments, Caterson noted that the omega-3s also blocked the activity of tumor necrosis factor alpha, a powerful inflammation-promoting compound.

Fish Oils Help in Rheumatoid Arthritis, Too

In a study reported in the May 2008 issue of *Rheumatology*, doctors asked ninety-seven patients to take either 10 grams of cod liver oil daily (providing 2.2 grams of omega-3s) or placebos for nine months. About 40 percent of patients taking the cod liver oil were able to reduce their use of nonsteroidal anti-inflammatory drugs (NSAIDs) by one-third or more during the course of the study. This was good news for two reasons: One, although the researchers did not directly measure pain or flexibility in the patients, less dependence on NSAIDs reflects less pain. Two, taking fewer NSAIDs reduces the risk of experiencing drug complications, including gastric ulcers and compromised liver function.

—⁓—

Discussing Nutritional and Herbal Supplements with Your Physician

If you are like many people, you have been frustrated when you tried to discuss supplements with your physician. All too often, doctors quickly dismiss their patients' questions about supplements.

Why? Nobel laureate and vitamin advocate Linus Pauling, Ph.D., explained it this way: "If a doctor isn't 'up' on something, he's 'down' on it." That is *really* the case.

Unfortunately, most physicians don't know much about nutrition because medical schools have given the subject a very low priority. Medicine, as the name suggests, places the greatest emphasis on pharmaceutical medicines and surgery. Furthermore, it's difficult for many people, including physicians, to admit that they don't know much about a particular subject. How often do you hear anyone admit, "I don't know much about that?"

Many physicians' critical thinking processes tend to be very narrow, and doctors can be as gullible as anyone in the world at large, swayed by the limitations of their own training, pharmaceutical company advertising, and misleading articles that question the value of diet and vitamin supplements.

The nutritionally oriented physicians whom I know suggest that the best way to talk about nutritional therapies with a skeptical doctor is to be firm but nonconfrontational. Physicians don't have a lot of time to keep up with their specialties, let alone delve into another one, such as nutrition. They may also have financial and therapeutic constraints imposed by health maintenance organizations (HMOs), insurers, or even the other doctors in their offices or hospitals, limiting what they can actually do in terms of treatment.

So, one approach might be to say something like, "Doctor, using vitamins, fatty acids, and herbs to reduce my inflammation appeals to me because they are safe and the evidence seems pretty solid. I would prefer not to treat myself, so, as your patient, I would like you to take some time to seriously study some of the research in this area. I'll even lend you this book. Please do me a favor and take the time to look into this and work with me."

If a sincere appeal fails, you may have to change physicians in order to find one who is nutritionally oriented or "integrative." This is easier than it used to be, and the names of several organizations that make referrals of nutritionally oriented doctors are listed in the appendix at www.inflammationsyndrome.com. Most nutritionally oriented physicians are not part of HMOs, and insurers may reimburse for only some of their services. In other words, they work in a traditional fee-for-service arrangement, so you will have to pay yourself. This may be more expensive, but it will likely lead to you gaining a nutritional program, a doctor who takes a little more time with you, and better care. You might be able to get mediocre care for free, but is that what you really want for your long-term health?

—m—

Fish Oils May Reduce Cancer Risk

Eating foods that are rich in omega-3 fatty acids or taking fish oil supplements may reduce the risk of developing cancer. Bruce N. Ames, Ph.D., an eminent cell biologist at the University of California, Berkeley, noted that 30 percent of cancers result from chronic inflammation or chronic infections. (Infections increase inflammation.)

The benefits of omega-3s are most striking in breast and prostate cancers. Studies have found that large amounts of linoleic acid (the parent omega-6 molecule) in corn oil and other common cooking oils increase the proliferation of breast and prostate cancer cells. In contrast, fish oils can prevent and slow the growth of these cancers. Corn oil has an omega-6 to omega-3 ratio of 60:1, and safflower oil a ratio of 77:1—far from our ancient balance of 1:1.

Some of the omega-6 fatty acids, particularly arachidonic acid, activate a variety of pro-inflammatory compounds, such as nuclear factor kappa beta (NFkB). NFkB activates genes involved in inflammation, and it also stimulates the activity of cancer cells. The omega-3 fatty acids (and many antioxidants) dampen the activity of NFkB.

Human studies have been consistent with cell and animal studies showing that omega-3 fish oils reduce the risk of developing cancer. Paul Terry, Ph.D., and his colleagues at the Karolinska Institute in Sweden tracked the health of more than 6,000 male twins, beginning when most of the men were in their midfifties. Terry found that men who regularly ate fish had one-half to one-third the risk of getting prostate cancer, compared with those who did not eat fish.

Fish Oils Improve Mood

There is growing evidence that inflammation in the brain is related to many diseases, including multiple sclerosis, and that inflammation of the tissues or the blood vessels in the brain affects our moods. The reason is that psychological stress increases the body's production of pro-inflammatory molecules.

Between 50 and 60 percent of the brain consists of fat, and the types of fat in your brain tend to reflect your eating habits. EPA and DHA get incorporated into the fatty membranes (walls) of cells, where they influence how cells communicate with one another. When other fats are incorporated in their place, communication between brain cells is disrupted.

In ancient times, people consumed roughly equal amounts of the omega-3s and the omega-6s and no trans fats. Today, the average American consumes twenty to thirty times more omega-6s than omega-3s, as well as substantial amounts of trans fats. As a result, the omega-3s are virtually nonexistent in many people's diets, contributing to depression and other mood disorders.

A high intake of the omega-6s increases the risk of suffering from depression, whereas many studies have found that omega-3 fish oil supplements are helpful in treating depression. These studies have included both children and adults and have shown that 2 to 6 grams of fish oils daily is a beneficial amount to take.

Supplements of the omega-3s can help reduce impulsive behavior, hostility, and physical aggressiveness. For example, a double-blind study of forty middle-age men and women found that 1.5 grams of DHA daily led to significant reductions in aggressive behavior in only two months. Meanwhile, when prison inmates in England were given fish oil supplements, their behavior improved and they were far less likely to act violently.

The mood and cognitive benefits of eating fish and taking fish oil supplements pay off in the long run, too. Numerous studies have found that people who regularly eat fish or take fish oil supplements maintain better memories as they age and are less likely to develop cognitive problems and Alzheimer's disease.

Fish Oils Protect the Eyes

Several studies have found that the omega-3s can reduce the risk of age-related macular degeneration (AMD), the leading cause of blindness among seniors. Researchers at the University of Melbourne, Australia, analyzed nine studies that focused on fish consumption and omega-3 intake in relation to AMD. People who ate fish at least twice each week had a one-fourth lower risk of developing early-onset AMD and a one-third lower risk of having late-onset AMD. A high intake of omega-3 fatty acids from all sources was associated with almost a 40 percent lower risk of developing AMD.

The incidence of AMD also rises when people's diets are low in lutein, an antioxidant found in spinach, kale, broccoli, and other dark green vegetables. Lutein forms the macular pigment, a yellowish region in the center of the eye's retina. Supplements increase the thickness of the macular pigment, and a combination of lutein and DHA seems to be particularly beneficial to the eyes. Researchers at Tufts University, Boston, found that taking 12 mg of lutein and 800 mg of DHA supplements improved the macular pigment but in slightly different ways. The lutein supplements increased the thickness of the outer region of the macular pigment, whereas the DHA supplements thickened the central part of the macular pigment.

Another study, conducted at Harvard University, found that a high intake of omega-3 fatty acids reduced the incidence of dry eyes, whereas a low intake of omega-3 fatty acids increased the occurrence. A high intake of omega-6 fatty acids, particularly linoleic acid, seemed to heighten the chances of developing dry eyes.

Fish Oils May Help with Weight Loss

The types of fats you consume influence weight gain and loss, regardless of their calories, and omega-3 fish oils may help you lose weight. In effect, fish oils appear to counteract the tendency of trans fats to increase body fat.

Researchers at the University of South Australia, Adelaide, asked study participants to take various supplements, including 1,560 mg of DHA and 360 mg of EPA daily, and to engage in light exercise for three months. The combination of fish oils and exercise led to each person experiencing several pounds of weight loss—more than with people taking a placebo and exercising.

The Problem with Flaxseed Oil

Some companies market flaxseed oil as an alternative to omega-3 fish oils. Flax may have some health benefits, but it is not a reliable source of

EPA and DHA. Flaxseed oil contains only alpha-linolenic acid and no EPA and DHA.

The idea is that your body will convert the alpha-linolenic acid in flaxseed oil to EPA and DHA. This conversion, however, is fraught with problems. First, most people do not accomplish this conversion with great efficiency. Sometimes the reason is related to age: older people have more difficulty with the conversion. A more common problem is that trans fats disable the delta-6-desaturase enzyme, which is crucial to the conversion. Even if you currently avoid foods containing trans fats, you likely ate them at some point over the last thirty years and your body may have lasting damage from them.

If you are a vegetarian and don't consume fish, you may think that flaxseed oil is your only option. Again, it is not equivalent to fish oils. Some companies, however, are preparing to market echium oil supplements, derived from *Echium plantagineum*, a plant that contains both gamma-linolenic acid and stearidonic acid. The delta-6-desaturase enzyme converts alpha-linolenic acid to stearidonic acid but not very efficiently. Yet studies have shown that people do readily convert stearidonic acid to EPA.

Three Recommended Supplements

As your first step to reducing inflammation, I recommend taking omega-3 fish oils (which contain EPA and DHA) and gamma-linolenic acid (GLA). You'll find many different brands on the market, but these are the three I recommend.

1. *Carlson Inflammation Balance.* This is my top recommendation; a high-potency combination of EPA, DHA, and GLA. These three fatty acids are the building blocks of the body's most powerful anti-inflammatory compounds. The product contains 200 mg of omega-3 fatty acids (EPA and DHA) and 200 mg of GLA per capsule. You can take one to three capsules daily. It's difficult to find combinations like this, and consumers can safely increase the daily number of capsules to suit their personal needs. Inflammation Balance contains 1,000 IU of vitamin D and 100 IU of vitamin E per capsule, as well, which also have anti-inflammatory benefits. (More details can be found at www.carlsonlabs.com.) *Tip*: Start by taking four capsules daily for two weeks to rapidly increase the concentration of these fatty acids in your body, then try reducing the amount to

two capsules daily. Consider adding a multi-antioxidant formula as well, such as Carlson's Aces or Aces Elite for even greater anti-inflammatory benefits.

2. *Carlson Very Finest Fish Oil*. This liquid fish oil (flavored with a hint of lemon or orange) provides 800 mg of EPA and 500 mg of DHA per teaspoon. Unlike other fish oil products, this one actually tastes good because of the slight lemon or orange flavor. Carlson sells a range of fish oil, salmon oil, and cod liver oil products in liquid and capsule form. (More details can be found at www.carlsonlabs.com.)

3. *Solgar Super GLA*. This is a high-potency supplement containing 300 mg of GLA per capsule. Many people benefit from large amounts of GLA, which can boost the anti-inflammatory activity of omega-3 fatty acids. The capsules have a slight citrus flavor and can be chewed. (More details can be found at www.solgar.com.)

How to Use Omega-3 Fish Oil Supplements

With all of the fish oil supplements on the market, it can be difficult to decide which brand to buy. As a general rule, I suggest that you opt for a brand that harvests fish from relatively pollution-free waters, such as those off the west coast of Norway. Some omega-3 supplements are derived from salmon, whereas others come from smaller fish, such as sardines and anchovies. Analyses by an independent testing laboratory (www.consumerlab.com) found that all of the omega-3 fish oil supplements tested were free of mercury. The mercury and other likely contaminants are removed during the extraction and refining of the fish oils.

Various fish oil supplements contain different ratios of EPA and DHA, with some being higher in EPA and others higher in DHA. Although EPA seems to have greater anti-inflammatory benefits, DHA should not be ignored. DHA promotes the production of resolvins and protectins, which have tremendous anti-inflammatory benefits, even though the body makes them in tiny quantities.

To reduce the risk of developing coronary heart disease and other inflammatory disorders, take at least 1 gram of omega-3 fish oil capsules daily. In most cases, this will be a single capsule. If you have any type of arthritis, take at least 3 grams daily and strive to eat coldwater fish (e.g., salmon, tuna, herring) once or twice a week. If you are taking a blood-thinning drug, such as aspirin or Coumadin, check with your physician because fish oils may further thin your blood.

Nelda: Fish Oil to Relieve Pain

At age sixty-three, Nelda displayed all the signs of rheumatoid arthritis. Her fingers, which hurt all the time, had become red and deformed. She was taking prescription pain relievers six to eight times daily, and her family physician suggested that it might be better to replace her right knee and left hip joints. Nelda was also taking nitroglycerin for her heart and a blood pressure–lowering medication.

She figured there had to be an alternative, so she visited Hugh D. Riordan, M.D., the president of the Center for the Improvement of Human Functioning International in Wichita, Kansas. Laboratory tests showed Nelda to be sensitive to some of her favorite foods, specifically dairy products and white potatoes, which she immediately stopped eating. She also began to take a number of anti-inflammatory supplements, including fish oils and antioxidant vitamins.

In less than a year Nelda was virtually pain-free and had regained flexibility in her fingers. She stood straight and no longer needed a cane or a walker. For the next twenty years Nelda remained active, healthier in her seventies and eighties than in her sixties.

Gamma-Linolenic Acid

Gamma-linolenic acid (GLA) is often misunderstood and undervalued for its anti-inflammatory benefits. Although GLA is part of the omega-6 family, it supports anti-inflammatory compounds in parallel with the omega-3s.

GLA supplements leapfrog the biochemical bottleneck caused by a weak or defective delta-6-desaturase enzyme, which would normally convert linoleic acid to GLA. The body quickly converts the GLA in supplements to dihomo-gamma-linolenic acid (DGLA), which is the "activated" form of GLA. At this point, DGLA can be converted either to pro-inflammatory arachidonic acid or to anti-inflammatory prostaglandin E_1. Meanwhile, EPA slows production of arachidonic acid, so as a consequence, GLA and DGLA further increase the activity of prostaglandin E_1. It's important to remember the synergism of GLA and EPA—they have greater anti-inflammatory benefits together than either does by itself.

Because GLA supports the anti-inflammatory effects of prostaglandin E_1, it inhibits several promoters of inflammation, including tumor necrosis factor alpha, interleukin-1 beta, and the abnormal proliferation of immune cells. Although the research on GLA might at times strike you as "miraculous," particularly with respect to its benefits in the treatment of brain cancer, all of the benefits are actually related to correcting and improving the body's metabolism of essential fats.

GLA Reduces Symptoms of Rheumatoid Arthritis

Several studies on people have found that GLA supplements dampen the destructive auto-immune activity that is characteristic of rheumatoid arthritis. In one of the clinical trials, Robert Zurier, M.D., of the University of Massachusetts, Worcester, treated thirty-seven patients with rheumatoid arthritis. He gave them either 1.4 grams of GLA or placebos daily for twenty-four weeks. By the end of the study, patients taking GLA had a 36 percent reduction in tender joints, and their overall score on tests measuring joint pain decreased by 45 percent.

The patients experienced other benefits as well. Overall, their number of swollen joints decreased by 28 percent, and the patients' overall score for swollen joints fell by 41 percent. Some people benefited far more than did others, but that is often the case with single-nutrient studies. It is likely that a broader supplement regimen (including the omega-3s) would have led to even more improvements.

In another study, Zurier doubled the dosage of GLA, giving fifty-six patients either 2.8 grams daily of the supplement or placebos for six months. This higher dosage led to significant improvements—at least a 25 percent improvement in four of eight measures of rheumatoid arthritis severity. For a second six-month period, Zurier gave GLA to all of the patients, and improvements were noted across the board. The group that was originally given GLA continued to improve over the course of a full year, with more than three-fourths of the patients experiencing decreased arthritic symptoms.

GLA Eases Injuries and Inflammation

The synergism of GLA and the omega-3 fish oils has been clearly demonstrated by Søren Mavrogenis, the physical therapist for the Danish Olympic team. Since 1996, he has used high doses of both oils to treat Olympians and other elite athletes with inflammatory overuse injuries. (See an additional discussion on pages 139–140 and 203–204.) But the benefits also extend to average people, "weekend warrior" athletes, and others who occasionally overexert themselves.

Mavrogenis has used GLA and fish oils to treat hundreds of patients. In a study published in the journal *Physical Therapy in Sport*, he focused on forty recreational athletes who took either placebos or a proprietary combination of 640 mg of omega-3 fatty acids, 672 mg of GLA, and small amounts of antioxidants for one month. All of the subjects suffered from some type of tendonitis related to athletic injuries, and they also received physical therapy.

By the end of the month, people who took the supplements had an almost complete recovery from pain, and they were able to continue exercising during the treatment. Mavrogenis noted that most patients recovered within two to three weeks, although people with more severe injuries may take as long as two months.

GLA Is Helpful in Eliminating Psoriasis and Eczema

The skin contains a reservoir of fatty acids, which serves partly as a barrier that protects against moisture loss. In fact, one of the classic signs of a fatty-acid deficiency is dry skin. Studies have found that other skin problems, such as psoriasis and eczema, may be resolved with supplements of GLA. It is likely that a combination of GLA and omega-3 fish oils will yield even greater benefits.

Swiss researchers gave forty men and women supplements containing 345 mg of GLA or placebos daily for twelve weeks. Over the course of the study, the subjects' skin moisture, firmness, elasticity, and smoothness improved. A number of studies have looked at whether GLA might reduce eczema and psoriasis. Although the results were not entirely consistent, the beneficial amount of GLA tended to be 275 mg or more daily. Adding omega-3 fish oils and vitamin D will likely lead to greater improvements.

Joan: Vitamins and Psoriasis

Since her early twenties, Joan had suffered from psoriasis, which doctors treated with limited success over the years with a variety of medications. At age fifty-six, she consulted Richard P. Huemer, M.D., a nutritionally oriented physician in Lancaster, California. Huemer confirmed the original diagnosis of psoriasis, based on her characteristic skin lesions, measleslike rashing, and scaling.

He also diagnosed Joan with intestinal dysbiosis, which can result in myriad symptoms, including allergylike symptoms and skin disorders.

He recommended that Joan take digestive aid supplements, as well as vitamin C, vitamin E, and gamma-linolenic acid supplements. Huemer also suggested that she try homeopathic remedies, such as 6X graphites.

Joan's psoriasis improved over the next few months. After four months, she was pleased to report to Huemer that her friends had told her she no longer had any signs of psoriasis.

GLA May Help You Keep Off Excess Pounds

We know that trans fats interfere with the body's production of GLA and, as a consequence, promote the accumulation of fat around the belly. So, could GLA supplements correct the problem and help with weight loss? The answer is tentatively yes, based on a study of obese adults at the University of California, Davis.

Stephen D. Phinney, M.D., Ph.D., asked fifty obese patients, all of whom had recently lost substantial amounts of weight, to take either 890 mg of GLA or placebos daily for one year. Most of the patients taking GLA supplements regained far less weight than did those taking placebos. On average, people taking GLA supplements regained only 4 pounds, compared with an almost 17-pound weight gain among people taking placebos.

GLA May Have Therapeutic Benefits in Brain Cancer

The most innovative use of GLA is in the treatment of brain cancer, which is difficult to successfully treat with surgery or radiation. GLA's benefits may apply to other types of cancer as well. Having said this, I must add that GLA is a highly experimental therapy for brain cancer, and it does not appear to be available in U.S. hospitals.

In an article in *Medical Science Monitor*, Undurti N. Das, M.D., described cell, animal, and human studies in which GLA was used to treat various types of brain cancer. In the three human studies detailed by Das, GLA was injected directly into the brain tumors, with individual dosages of 0.5 to 1 mg and total dosages of GLA ranging from 4.5 to 20 mg over periods of up to twenty days. The GLA caused significant reductions in tumor size without the patients' experiencing significant side effects, and most of the patients were alive and well three years after their diagnoses (at the time that Das published his article). Survival was usually related to the size of the patient's tumor at the time of treatment.

In separate cell studies, researchers at the Northwestern University

School of Medicine, Chicago, found that GLA supplements can reduce the activity of Her-2, a gene that increases the aggressiveness of breast cancer. Women who have breast cancer and are also Her-2 positive are less likely to benefit from chemotherapy or hormone treatments to control cancer. GLA reduces Her-2 levels and, as a result, might improve the efficacy of other therapies.

How to Buy and Use GLA Supplements

GLA supplements are derived from borage, evening primrose, or black currant seeds. GLA constitutes about 20 percent of borage seed oil, 15 to 19 percent of black currant seed oil, and 9 percent of evening primrose oil. You may read that one source is better than another, but the plant source is not as important as the actual amount of GLA per capsule.

Many of the supplements are labeled "borage seed oil," "black currant seed oil," or "evening primrose oil," and some companies try to obscure the actual amount of GLA in their products. The reason is that the seed oils are relatively inexpensive, but producing higher concentrations of GLA gets progressively more expensive. It is not uncommon to find products that provide, as an example, 1,000 mg of evening primrose oil but only 50 mg of GLA. Read the fine print to see how much actual GLA is in each capsule. Then calculate the daily amount that you want and what it will cost you.

A daily GLA dose of 100 to 200 mg should be adequate for most people and, again, it is important to take both GLA and fish oil supplements for their dual anti-inflammatory benefits. If you are trying to resolve an acute anti-inflammatory condition, such as a soft tissue (tendon or muscle) injury, increase the amount to 300 to 600 mg daily, and then try lowering the dose after one month. If you have a more severe inflammatory disease, such as rheumatoid arthritis, strive for 1.4 to 2.8 grams (1,400 to 2,800 mg) daily, which is what the studies have found to be effective. You can likely achieve equal or greater benefits, however, with a smaller amount of GLA combined with omega-3 fish oils.

Victor: Olympic Nutrition

Søren Mavrogenis, the physiotherapist for the Danish Olympic team, began to recommend a combination of omega-3 fatty acids, gamma-linolenic acid, and antioxidants in 1996. At the time, he had been treating the inflamed knee of a female rower but had not been able to help her. Because of the side effects of nonsteroidal anti-inflammatory drugs (NSAIDs), Mavrogenis was reluctant to recommend them for long-term use.

Mavrogenis's conversations with health writer Bjørn Falck Madsen of Denmark and a researcher at a Scandinavian vitamin company led to his devising a specific supplement regimen. The rower started taking the supplements and was able to resume rowing within a few weeks. One success led to another, and today Mavrogenis routinely uses a combination of omega-3 fatty acids, gamma-linolenic acid, and antioxidants (brand name PharmaNord Bio-Sport), along with deep-muscle massage, to treat chronic overuse and inflammatory disorders. About one-third of his clinic's patients are elite athletes.

One of Mavrogenis's patients has been Victor A. Feddersen, a world-champion rower and an Olympic gold medalist in 1996. During training and competition, Feddersen suffered inflammatory injuries to his elbows. In the past he had to take a break from training and use NSAIDs. But for the last few years Feddersen has taken fatty acid and antioxidant supplements while also undergoing Mavrogenis's deep-muscle massage. It has made a big difference. Feddersen responds quickly to the supplements and has been able to continue training while he recuperates.

Other Danish Olympic athletes have benefited similarly with a variety of inflammatory injuries, including those of the shoulders, arms, legs, and Achilles' heel. In general, inflammation subsides about a month after the athletes start taking the supplements, but some people have responded within a week, while others need several months.

Olive Oil

Think of olive oil as one of the tastiest "supplements" you can eat. A common constituent of Greek and Italian diets, olive oil is rich in oleic acid, an omega-9 fatty acid. Many of the heart-healthy benefits of the traditional Mediterranean diet have been attributed to the abundant use of olive oil. Although other aspects of the diet (e.g., fruits, vegetables, and fish) are healthful, scientific studies have found olive oil to possess impressive anti-inflammatory properties in its own right.

Diets high in olive oil appear to reduce the likelihood of developing rheumatoid arthritis. Christos S. Mantzoros, M.D., D.Sc., of Harvard Medical School, and researchers from the Athens Medical School found that consumption of olive oil was associated with a 61 percent lower risk of having rheumatoid arthritis. In another study, Parveen Yaqoob, Ph.D., a researcher at the University of Southampton, England, asked healthy middle-age men to follow either a conventional diet or one high in olive oil for two months. The men consuming extra olive oil had a specific type of "adhesion molecule" that was 20 percent less active. This adhesion molecule, known as ICAM-1, sustains inflammatory and allergic reactions. By reducing the activity of adhesion molecules, olive oil tempers inflammatory reactions.

How to Buy and Use Olive Oil

As was discussed in chapter 6, the best varieties of olive oil are "extra virgin," because they are produced during the first mechanical pressing of olives. Pure or classic olive oil is also made from the first pressing, but it is slightly more acidic and can tolerate higher cooking temperatures. Light olive oil has been filtered to reduce its natural fragrance; it has no fewer calories than the other forms.

You should use olive oil exclusively or nearly exclusively as your cooking oil. Grapeseed oil is also rich in omega-9 fatty acids, but it is often produced through chemical extraction. Some mechanically pressed grapeseed oil is available, but you have to search for it in stores. While grapeseed oil is tolerant of very high temperatures, olive oil is still the preferred oil at home and in restaurants.

Other major food sources of omega-9 fatty acids are avocados and macadamia nuts. Both foods have been shown to reduce blood cholesterol levels, although their health benefits may be partly related to other nutrients.

In this chapter you have read how "good" fats can help restore a normal inflammatory response and, in doing so, reduce symptoms of rheumatoid arthritis, osteoarthritis, and other inflammatory disorders. These fats can also lower blood pressure and lessen your risk of developing heart disease and cancer. In the following chapter you will learn how various herbs are being used to fight inflammation.

CHAPTER 9

The Power of
Anti-Inflammatory
Herbs

Conventional medicine often dismisses the health benefits of medicinal and culinary (kitchen) herbs as unproven folk remedies. Herbs were our ancestors' original medicines, however, and evidence of their use has been found in 60,000-year-old burial sites. Today, herbal remedies remain extraordinarily popular throughout the world, and thousands of scientific studies document their benefits in alleviating a wide range of health problems.

Although many doctors will deny the therapeutic efficacy of herbs, almost 40 percent of all pharmaceutical drugs are based on molecules originally identified in plants. Aspirin, chemically known as acetylsalicylic acid, was originally used in the form of willow tree bark, which contains salicylic acid. Digitalis, a powerful heart stimulant, is still extracted from the leaves of foxglove because the compounds are too complex to synthesize.

Thanks to cell and molecular biologists, we now understand exactly why many herbs and other plant constituents have powerful anti-inflammatory and pain-reducing benefits. Although plants contain vitamins and minerals, most of their biological activity comes from antioxidant and anti-inflammatory compounds called polyphenolic flavonoids.

Herbal medicines are very different from pharmaceuticals. Most drugs consist of single synthetic compounds. In contrast, herbs possess unique combinations of multiple compounds that work in myriad ways. In fact, some plants contain hundreds of polyphenolic flavonoids, many of which provide anti-inflammatory benefits. Another difference: drugs have a high risk of producing side effects, whereas herbal remedies rarely cause side effects.

Herbs reduce inflammation through several mechanisms:

- By functioning as antioxidants that quench free radicals, thus putting the brakes on pro-inflammatory processes;
- By blocking the activity of Cox-2, one of the enzymes involved in producing inflammation-promoting compounds;
- By regulating and inhibiting pro-inflammatory chemicals, such as nuclear factor kappa beta and tumor necrosis factor alpha; and
- By turning off genes involved in inflammation, in effect shutting down an inflammatory response at the most basic level of our biology.

In this chapter I discuss three of my favorite anti-inflammatory herbs—curcumin, Pycnogenol, and boswellia—as well as several others.

Curcumin

The spice turmeric, obtained from the rhizome of *Curcuma longa*, has long been a staple in southeast Asian cuisine and in Ayurveda, India's traditional medicine system. About 3 percent of turmeric consists of several curcuminoids, which are generally referred to simply as curcumin. Curcumin has extremely powerful anti-inflammatory properties. The science is solid: more than 2,000 medical and scientific studies support the use of curcumin.

What distinguishes curcumin is its ability to reduce inflammation through at least ninety-seven different biological mechanisms, according to an article by Bharat B. Aggarwal, Ph.D., in *Biochemical Pharmacology*. For example, curcumin lessens the activity of interleukin-6, nuclear factor kappa beta, macrophage inflammatory protein, lipoxygenase, tumor necrosis factor alpha (TNF-a), matrix metalloproteinase, several types of protein kinases, adhesion molecules, and genes involved in inflammation. To date, no other substance has been discovered or developed with such far-reaching anti-inflammatory benefits.

Much of the research on curcumin has been conducted by Aggarwal and his colleagues at the University of Texas MD Anderson Cancer Treatment Center, in Houston. This center is widely regarded as the best conventional cancer treatment center in the United States. In the 1980s, Aggarwal discovered tumor necrosis factor alpha, a chemical released by the immune system that promotes both inflammation and the growth of cancers. As he searched for compounds to counter TNF-a's destructive properties, he began to study curcumin.

The list of diseases that curcumin helps is long—and growing—and includes rheumatoid arthritis, psoriasis, irritable bowel syndrome, colorectal polyps, and age-related cognitive impairment. By quenching the fires of inflammation, it's likely to help almost any disorder.

Rheumatoid arthritis. In a study conducted at the University of Arizona Health Sciences Center, Tucson, researchers used a curcumin-rich turmeric extract to treat rheumatoid arthritis in laboratory animals. The extract blocked joint inflammation and the breakdown of joint cartilage and bone. The researchers determined that curcumin worked by deactivating genes that promoted inflammation.

It's possible that curcumin has some synergism with the omega-3 fatty acids and gamma-linolenic acid because all three nutritional compounds reduce pro-inflammatory prostaglandin E_2. In a study of people, a single dose of 3.6 grams (3,600 mg) of curcumin reduced prostaglandin E_2 levels by two-thirds after only one hour. After study participants had consumed curcumin for one month, their PGE_2 levels remained 57 percent lower than before supplementation began.

Cancer. Patients with cancer have a strong undercurrent of inflammation, which likely encourages the proliferation of tumors. Curcumin holds tremendous promise in preventing cancer and when used in conjunction with other therapies. A variety of animal studies have found that curcumin can protect against colon, intestinal, oral, and skin cancers. Its benefits derive from several mechanisms. First, it blocks the life cycle of cancer cells, leading to cell destruction (apoptosis). It also quenches free radicals and inflammation, both of which can lead to cancer-causing cell mutations.

Two dozen human studies are currently under way to determine the added benefits of curcumin in the treatment of cancer. The dosages of curcumin in these studies range from 2 to 8 grams daily. Physicians and researchers at the MD Anderson Cancer Treatment Center recently published a study showing that large amounts of curcumin helped certain patients with pancreatic cancer, one of the deadliest forms of the disease; however, some anecdotal reports indicate that large amounts of curcumin may lead to the hemorrhaging of tumors, so consult your physician if you want to take more than 2 grams daily.

Alzheimer's disease. This form of dementia may result from the long-term inflammation of brain tissue. In a study described in the *American Journal of Epidemiology*, researchers determined that Singapore residents who made a regular habit of eating curry, which contains turmeric and other spices, had half the risk of developing cognitive problems in old age, compared with people who rarely ate curry. Even people who occasionally ate curry had a 38 percent lower risk of cognitive impairment. In India, where curry is practically the national dish, the prevalence of Alzheimer's disease among the elderly is one-fourth that of the United States.

Liver damage. Studies have found that curcumin can protect the liver against a variety of toxic compounds, which is important news for people suffering from inflammatory liver diseases, such as hepatitis or cirrhosis. Curcumin also reduced liver damage from aflatoxin, toxic chemicals, and excess iron. Another study found that curcumin inhibited the activation and spread of liver stellate cells, which play a role in the development of cirrhosis.

Ulcerative colitis. Inflammatory and irritable bowel diseases affect more than 5 million people in the United States. In Japan, doctors recently used curcumin, drugs, or placebos to treat 89 patients with ulcerative colitis. A combination of 2,000 mg curcumin daily and conventional medications led to the greatest benefits over six months of treatment.

Product recommendations. Two of my favorite curcumin supplements are CuraMed and Curamin, both manufactured by Terry Naturally (EuropharmaUSA.com, 866-598-5487). CuraMed contains a proprietary form of curcumin that its label says is equivalent to 4,000 mg of curcumin. Curamin contains a combination of curcumin, boswellia, and dl-phenylalanine, which act synergistically to reduce pain. Another interesting product from Terry Naturally is Arthocin, an herbal supplement formulated for people with joint and back pain. I also like Solgar's standardized Turmeric Root Extract (solgar.com), which yields 285 mg of curcumin per capsule.

Dorothy: Nutritional Supplements to Treat Cancer

Abram Hoffer, M.D., Ph.D., one of the pioneers in vitamin therapy, first began to treat cancer patients for depression and anxiety. He soon found that patients taking large dosages of vitamin C and other vitamins and minerals were living longer than those who did not. When his cases were analyzed by Nobel laureate Linus Pauling, Ph.D., it became clear that cancer patients lived several times longer (postdiagnosis) when they took supplements, compared with patients who chose not to take supplements.

Hoffer has treated more than 1,200 cancer patients since 1977, and some types of cancer (such as breast and prostate) are more responsive to supplements than other types (such as lung) are. One of his patients is Dorothy of Victoria, Canada.

Dorothy was first diagnosed with breast cancer when she was forty-nine years old and going through an emotionally draining divorce. Doctors performed a lumpectomy, gave her radiation therapy, and pronounced her treated and cured.

But conventional medicine didn't cure Dorothy. Her cancer eventually reappeared in one of her breasts and also spread to her lungs. For the last few years, however, Dorothy has been healthy and free of cancer. She credits her long-term survival to "quality" vitamin supplements, a good diet, and a great attitude toward life.

For many years, Dorothy took large amounts of vitamin A to reduce the risk of metastasis. The cancer did metastasize to her lungs twenty years after her initial diagnosis, however, but it receded after drug treatment.

In 1997, she consulted with Hoffer, and she has since been taking a high-powered assortment of nutritional supplements, including vitamins A, C, D, and E; beta-carotene; selenium; and vitaminlike coenzyme Q_{10}. "I do feel I need these extra supplements," Dorothy said. "I think anyone in this situation would need them."

Dorothy emphasizes organic foods in her diet, eating a lot of fish, vegetables, and occasionally game meats (deer, elk). Now in her mid-seventies, Dorothy is physically active, much more so than many other seniors who have not battled cancer. She soothes her soul and reduces stress with music, meditation, visualization, long walks, and a positive mental attitude.

Pycnogenol

Pycnogenol, an extract of French maritime pine bark (*Pinus pinaster*), is one of my favorite natural anti-inflammatory compounds. (I described my personal experience with Pycnogenol in the introduction.) Sometimes referred to as a complex of oligomeric proanthocyanidins, Pycnogenol is a patented complex of forty antioxidants. Research dating back to the 1930s found that flavonoids, similar to those in Pycnogenol, enhance the benefits of vitamin C in maintaining the integrity of blood vessel walls. A combination of vitamin C and Pycnogenol can reduce blood vessel fragility and leakage, which are often seen in people who experience unexplained bruising. A three-month study, published in *Redox Report*, found that Pycnogenol lowered CRP levels from 3.9 mg/L to 1.1 mg/L—a 72 percent decrease.

Inflammation. At dosages of 150 mg or higher daily, Pycnogenol has potent anti-inflammatory and pain-reducing benefits. A study in the August 2008 *Phytotherapy Research* found that Pycnogenol supplements lessened osteoarthritic knee pain by 40 percent and lowered overall osteoarthritis symptoms by 21 percent. Two out of every five patients were able to cut down their use of analgesic drugs.

Pycnogenol works in part by inhibiting the production of peroxides, which stimulate the inflammatory activity of white blood cells. For severe inflammation or pain, consider taking 300 mg of Pycnogenol daily. Pycnogenol impedes the activity of cyclooxygenase-2 (Cox-2), an enzyme known to promote inflammation. As a result, Pycnogenol appears to have broad anti-inflammatory properties. In children with asthma, Pycnogenol supplements led to improved lung function, and many of the children were able to reduce or stop using their medications.

Osteoarthritis. Several studies, including one published in *Nutrition Research*, found that Pycnogenol could alleviate pain and stiffness in people with osteoarthritis. The researchers asked patients to take 50 mg of Pycnogenol three times daily. After three months, the patients had an average reduction of 43 percent in pain and 35 percent in stiffness, along with a 52 percent improvement in physical function. In addition, the patients had less need for pain-relieving drugs.

Type 2 diabetes. The blood sugar abnormalities that are characteristic of type 2 diabetes promote inflammation, as does the excess weight typically associated with this condition. Pycnogenol supplements enhance glycemic control in people with diabetes. In one study, dosages ranging from 50 to 200 mg daily led to significant improvements in fasting glucose, postprandial glucose, and hemoglobin A_{1c}. In 2007, researchers reported that Pycnogenol blocks the activity of alpha-glucosidase, a carb-digesting enzyme. The mechanism is similar to that of the diabetes drug acarbose, but Pycnogenol is 190 times more potent than the drug in blocking alpha-glucosidase activity.

Cardiovascular health. Pycnogenol reduces the risk of developing cardiovascular disease. In one study, published in *Life Sciences*, researchers asked fifty-eight patients with high blood pressure to take 100 mg of Pycnogenol daily for twelve weeks. The supplements enhanced blood vessel tone, and many of the patients were able to safely reduce their dosage of medications that were used to treat hypertension. Other research has found that taking Pycnogenol supplements led to modest reductions in the "bad" low-density lipoprotein cholesterol and increases in the "good" high-density lipoprotein cholesterol.

Erectile dysfunction. The inability to achieve or maintain an erection is often a sign of cardiovascular disease, and men with erectile dysfunction are frequently diagnosed with heart disease within several years after the onset of erectile problems. The cardiovascular benefits of Pycnogenol extend to resolving erectile dysfunction in men. Researchers asked forty men to take Prelox, a proprietary combination of Pycnogenol and L-arginine (a protein building block). More than three-fourths of the men gained improvements in erectile function. L-arginine is the precursor to nitric oxide, a substance that regulates blood-vessel tone and the ability of blood-vessel walls to dilate (which is needed to maintain an erection).

Grape-seed extracts are also rich in proanthocyanidins, although their antioxidant constituents are somewhat different from those found in Pycnogenol. Grape-seed extracts have a similar strengthening effect on blood-vessel walls, and they possess anti-inflammatory properties as well. Some physicians have told me that patient responses are often individualized, with some responding better to either Pycnogenol or grape-seed extracts. One of the potential problems with grape-seed extracts is that there is less chemical consistency between batches.

Product recommendations. Although Pycnogenol is obtained from a single source in France, dozens of companies sell Pycnogenol supplements. Dosages and forms (capsules or tablets) will vary, as will price. I recommend Solgar's 100-mg Pycnogenol capsules.

Boswellia

Boswellia is the common name for the resins of *Boswellia serrata*, a tree that grows in India. The resins, also known as frankincense, have long been used in traditional Ayurvedic medicine, and they are rich in a group of anti-inflammatory compounds called boswellic acids.

This herbal extract is distinguished from other herbal compounds by its mode of action. Boswellia inhibits 5-lipoxygenase, one of the enzymes needed for the body's production of inflammatory compounds. It also blocks the activation of "complement," a type of inflammatory response. Although complement is an essential part of our immune defenses, its overactivity can contribute to chronic inflammation.

In several studies, participants have used 200 mg of boswellic acid extracts three times daily to treat rheumatoid arthritis, osteoarthritis, and associated inflammation. These studies have shown a reduction in symptoms, such as pain and morning stiffness, as well as in inflammatory markers. Preliminary research also suggests that boswellia may ease asthma.

A proprietary extract of boswellia known as 5-Loxin can significantly reduce symptoms of knee osteoarthritis, according to a study by American and Indian researchers. Siba R. Raychaudhuri, M.D., of the University of California School of Medicine, Davis, and colleagues treated seventy patients with 100 mg of 5-Loxin, 250 mg of 5-Loxin, or placebos daily for three months. Both doses of 5-Loxin led to significant reductions in pain and improvement in physical mobility and functioning; however, people taking the higher dose of 5-Loxin responded faster—within a week—and with greater improvements. The 5-Loxin extract also lowered levels of the enzyme matrix metalloproteinase-3 in the synovial fluid of subjects' knees. This enzyme is involved in the breakdown of cartilage. In the study, people taking placebos experienced no improvement.

Ginger

Few spices besides ginger root are versatile enough to flavor both entrées and desserts, from Asian meals to gingerbread cookies. Native to South Asia, ginger (*Zingiber officinale*) has become a popular spice around the world.

A close botanical relative of turmeric, ginger is rich in kaempferol, an antioxidant that inhibits the Cox-2 enzyme. Ginger also blocks lipoxygenase, another enzyme involved in the body's production of inflammatory compounds. It addition, it appears to contain trace amounts of melatonin, a hormone otherwise made by the pineal gland that has antioxidant and anti-inflammatory properties.

Both ginger and ginger-containing supplements have been found helpful in treating osteoarthritis, rheumatism, and muscular pain. Ginger has the added benefit of reducing morning sickness and motion sickness. Although you can take ginger supplements, I recommend adding it to your food. Ginger is common in grocery stores, but the best form (and the most difficult to find) is fresh baby ginger root, which is especially tender.

In a study published in the *American Journal of Obstetrics and*

Gynecology, researchers analyzed the findings of five studies in which ginger supplements were used to treat nausea following surgery. They found that taking 1 gram or more of ginger reduced nausea and vomiting by about one-third during the first day after surgery. A separate group of researchers proved that ingesting a combination of 1,000 mg of powdered ginger root, twice daily, along with a protein-rich drink, eased the nausea associated with chemotherapy.

—⁂—

Try This Anti-Inflammatory Tea

A British herb company, Pukka Herbs, has a "three ginger" blend of organic ginger, galangal, and golden turmeric. These three related herbs combine to make a potent yet safe anti-inflammatory tea, which you can enjoy hot or iced. Pukka Herbs recently began selling its teas in the United States. Some of my other favorites include the company's "three mint" and "detox" tea blends. If you're in the United States, visit www.healthmattersamerica.com or call (800) 304-1497. If you're in Europe, go to www.pukkaherbs.com.

—⁂—

Digestive Enzymes

Digestive enzymes, such as bromelain and papain derived from plants and trypsin and chymotrypsin made from animal sources, have been used to treat a variety of health problems, from arthritis to cancer. The quest to discover a specific mechanism to explain their benefits has been prolonged, although several theories may account for at least part of their effects.

Digestive enzymes break down food proteins, and undigested food proteins may trigger inflammatory reactions. These enzymes might also help break down infectious bacteria (in the gut), another trigger of inflammatory reactions. In addition, digestive enzymes may help regulate the immune system and, by enhancing cell-to-cell communication, they could turn off some of the genes involved in inflammation. Indeed, the body's largest group of immune cells lies in the gastrointestinal tract, intermingled with our digestive enzymes.

Product recommendations. You'll find dozens of digestive enzyme supplements on the market, but I recommend two specific products that have been used for more than forty years. One is Carlson's Digestive Aid #34, and the other is Wobbenzyme N. A probiotic (containing "good" intestinal bacteria) called Bio K+ might also have benefits, although it is not a digestive enzyme per se.

Resveratrol

Resveratrol (pronounced res-vair-uh-traul), an antioxidant found in small amounts in purple grapes, red wine, blueberries, and other plants, was first isolated from plants in 1940 but didn't attract much attention until the 1990s. Resveratrol is distinguished by its ability to promote health or longevity in a wide range of animals, from microscopic worms to human beings. In animal studies, resveratrol lengthened life expectancy, which is important because inflammation increases with aging.

Resveratrol works in large part by enhancing the activity of Sirt1, a gene that plays a central role in the longevity of numerous species, including humans. By boosting Sirt1 activity, resveratrol reduces the risk of developing age-related diseases, such as diabetes, heart disease, and cancer. Unfortunately, almost all of the research has been done in test tubes, yeast, worms, fruit flies, fish, and mice—not on people. That said, the single human study with resveratrol found promising benefits.

Anti-Aging. In studies conducted at Harvard University, mice that received supplemental resveratrol had higher activity of the Sirt1 gene. They also had lower levels of insulinlike growth factor-1, which is involved in inflammation and is also considered a risk factor for cancer. Furthermore, the mice lived about 15 percent longer—the equivalent of eleven human years—compared with mice that had a resveratrol-free diet. Even with advancing age, the mice maintained physical activity and coordination that were more like the abilities of younger mice. The benefits were all the more striking because the mice were fed the equivalent of a junk-food diet.

Diabetes. The Harvard University researchers found that mice eating a high-calorie diet and taking resveratrol did not develop diabetes; however, animals that did not get the antioxidant did develop the disease. In a small study of men with type 2 diabetes, resveratrol supplements reduced their fasting blood sugar levels and improved their insulin function, which is significant because diabetes accelerates the aging process. Additional human studies using resveratrol are under way.

Heart disease. Resveratrol may lower the risk of developing heart disease through a number of mechanisms. First, its anti-inflammatory properties may prevent or lessen damage to the arteries. Second, resveratrol may prevent the oxidation of cholesterol, which is regarded as an early step in the development of heart disease. Third, resveratrol has a mild blood-thinning effect, which would reduce the risk of developing blood clots.

Cancer. Although the research is experimental and based on cell and animal studies, growing evidence does suggest that resveratrol might have a role in cancer prevention. These studies have focused primarily on breast, prostate, liver, and pancreatic cancers. Resveratrol seems to prevent different stages of cancer growth and appears to reduce cell division and metastasis, according to an article in *Cell Cycle*. Seven studies that use resveratrol as an adjunct in treating people with cancer are under way, but the results won't be known for several years.

Product recommendations. Resveratrol supplements were originally extracted from grape skins, a by-product of the wine-making process. Most resveratrol supplements now come from Japanese knotweed (*Polygonum cuspidatum*), a less expensive source. I recommend Solgar's resveratrol products, called PC Extend in the United States and Resveratrol in Europe, as well as Solgar's Assist Plus, which contains a combination of resveratrol and pomegranate.

Cynthia: Antioxidants to Treat Hepatitis

At age thirty-three, Cynthia had received a blood transfusion following the birth of her daughter. Several weeks later, she developed a general sense of fatigue, along with muscle pains and jaundice. She quickly became too sick to care for her daughter.

Laboratory tests indicated that Cynthia had contracted hepatitis C, and her physician noted that the virus had also damaged her pancreas, resulting in elevated blood sugar levels and diabetes. Her prognosis was poor, but a specialist suggested that she have injections of interferon and antiviral drugs, which would result in her experiencing flulike symptoms for about six months. In addition, Cynthia was told that she would eventually need a liver transplant.

Seeking an alternative to interferon therapy and a liver transplant, Cynthia consulted with Burton M. Berkson, M.D., Ph.D., of Las Cruces, New Mexico. At the time, she was fatigued and her liver was enlarged and tender. Tests indicated that her liver enzymes were very high, and her fasting blood sugar level was 300 mg/dl (optimal is 75–85 mg/dl).

Berkson started Cynthia on his "triple antioxidant" approach, which included 600 mg of alpha-lipoic acid, 400 mcg of selenium, and 900 mg of silymarin daily. He also asked her to follow a diet similar to the AI Diet Plan, which was rich in protein and vegetables and low in refined carbohydrates. After two weeks, she had an increase in energy and resumed many normal activities. By the sixth week of supplementation, Cynthia's liver enzymes had fallen to near normal levels and her fasting glucose was 112 mg/dl. She has been following the diet and supplement regimen for more than five years and reports that she still feels great.

Other Natural Anti-Inflammatory Supplements

Many other natural products have impressive anti-inflammatory properties. Some, such as pomegranate and garlic, can be consumed as foods or supplements. Others, such as chamomile, are best taken as a tea. It may be difficult to choose among these nutrients and herbs, but you might find yourself benefiting from one or more of them.

Devil's claw. This herb (*Harpagophytum procumbens*), originally from southern Africa, can benefit people with rheumatoid arthritis, lower back pain, and various other rheumatic complaints. In one study, French researchers gave 435 mg of devil's claw daily to ninety-two people with osteoarthritis. By the end of the four-month study, people taking devil's claw had significantly less pain and greater mobility and also used fewer anti-inflammatory drugs and painkillers.

Cat's claw. Despite a similar common name, cat's claw (*Uncaria tomentosa*) is not related to devil's claw. Native to South America, cat's claw is known as una de gato. The herb's anti-inflammatory properties derive from its ability to inhibit the activity of nuclear factor kappa beta.

Chamomile. Brewed as a tea, chamomile (*Matricaria chamomilla*) has long been used in Europe to settle upset tummies. It has impressive anti-inflammatory properties and is sometimes an ingredient in cosmetics, such as those manufactured by Camo-Care. It may be of benefit in treating rashes and other skin problems.

Green tea. A particularly rich source of antioxidants, green tea (*Camellia sinensis*) contains epigallocatechin-3 gallate (EGCG), epigallocatechin (EGC), and epicatechin-3 gallate (ECG), which together form about 30 percent of the dry weight of tea leaves. Scores of studies by Japanese researchers have shown that green tea has anti-inflammatory benefits that may reduce the risk of developing heart disease and cancer.

High-quality green tea has an added bonus: it is rich in the amino acid L-theanine, which promotes mental focus and a sense of relaxation.

Garlic. This common condiment is rich in sulfur and selenium, two compounds that help maintain normal immune function. Garlic (*Allium sativum*) contains many compounds that are closely related to N-acetylcysteine, a powerful antioxidant that helps fight infections and reduces inflammation. The sulfur content of garlic enhances the production of glutathione, the most powerful antioxidant made by the body; the selenium in garlic enables the production of glutathione peroxidase, which helps the body break down toxins. I recommend that people include garlic in their meals, but aged garlic extracts (sold as Kyolic) are the best researched form of garlic supplements.

Quercetin. This antioxidant flavonoid is found in apples and onions, and it has excellent anti-inflammatory benefits, particularly in dealing with pollen allergies. It inhibits the activity of adhesion molecules, which promote many types of inflammatory reactions. Quercetin (pronounced kwair-sih-tin) is similar in chemical structure to cromolyn sodium (NasalCrom), a synthetic flavonoid drug that is used to prevent pollen allergies.

—⟊—

Jack's Herbal Tea

To reduce the upper-respiratory symptoms of colds and sore throats, as well as to calm upset tummies, I often recommend a tasty home-brewed tea. In a small pot or mug, steep two tea bags, one containing chamomile and the other with either peppermint or spearmint. Add one-half to one teaspoon of dried rose hips and steep. Before serving, remove the tea bags and the rose hips (strain, if necessary) and sweeten the tea with a small amount of honey.

—⟊—

CHAPTER 10

The Anti-Inflammatory Benefits of a Multivitamin Supplement

The previous two chapters focused on specific supplements that quell the intense fires of inflammation. Yet good nutrition is more than the simple sum of nutrients. In this chapter, I focus on the many benefits of taking multivitamin and multimineral supplements.

There are countless good reasons to take a multivitamin and multimineral supplement. The chief reason is to reduce the risk of developing nutrient deficiencies, caused by poor eating habits, other harmful lifestyle behaviors, or higher-than-normal individual requirements. According to data from the U.S. Department of Agriculture, vitamin and mineral deficiencies are common: 81 percent of Americans do not consume the Daily Reference Intake (DRI, formerly the Recommended Dietary Allowance) of vitamin E, 75 percent do not have enough folic acid in their diets, 54 percent do not consume sufficient vitamin A, and roughly 20 to 33 percent of Americans fail to get enough B vitamins. If you consider that the DRIs are conservative recommendations, the prevalence of deficiencies is even worse. Furthermore, most medications interfere with nutrient absorption or utilization. For example, acid-reducing drugs lower the absorption of vitamins B_{12} and C, oral contraceptives reduce the levels of most of the B vitamins, and statins block the body's production of vitaminlike coenzyme Q_{10}.

A multivitamin and multimineral supplement can close the gap between marginal intakes or outright deficiencies and more optimal intake. A study in the *Journal of the American Dietetic Association* found that only half of middle-age and older men and women obtained the recommended amounts of vitamins and minerals from their diets; however, 80 percent of them did subsequently achieve the recommended amounts when they took vitamin and mineral supplements.

A multivitamin and multimineral supplement can also help protect against inflammation. Low levels or deficiencies of some nutrients can affect the body's ability to regulate inflammation and may even stimulate inflammation. For example, an inadequate intake of zinc can increase levels of free radicals, which promote inflammation, and a lack of magnesium heightens your susceptibility to free radical damage. In addition, some of the B vitamins serve as cofactors in antioxidant activities, again helping to lessen inflammation.

In fact, several studies have found that multivitamins can reduce levels of C-reactive protein, an important marker of inflammation. Like

Percentage of Americans <u>Not</u> Meeting the Government's Recommended Daily Intakes of Vitamins and Minerals

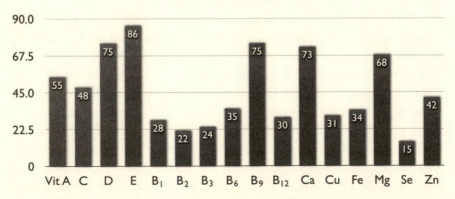

Based on USDA data at www.ars.usda.gov/Services/docs.htm?docid=10709 and Ginde, A. A. *Archives of Internal Medicine*, 2009;169:626–632.

other types of supplements, a multivitamin can have many "side bene-fits." Some research has shown that multivitamins improve mood, and they can also cut the rate of DNA damage, which is important for lower-ing the risk of developing cancer.

In addition, a multivitamin can simplify a big part of your supple-ment regimen. You can certainly take a dozen different supplements each day, but even if you can afford to do so, you may have difficulty staying with such a program because of the hassle of counting out all of the cap-sules and the tablets. As an example, if you take a multivitamin, a fish oil capsule, and a curcumin supplement, this can reduce the number of pills to three to four.

I typically recommend vitamin brands that are sold in health food or natural food stores. As a general rule, they have higher, more biologically active potencies, compared with the more popular drugstore brands. Drugstore brands of once-a-day multivitamins tend to contain 100 per-cent of the DRI, an amount that is woefully inadequate for most people. DRI levels might prevent the most serious types of vitamin deficiencies, but they do not contribute to a more optimal nutritional intake. This is why I recommend a *high-potency* multivitamin; as a guideline, look for daily doses of 20 to 50 mg of vitamins B_1, B_2, B_3, and B_6. Another advan-tage of health food brands: they almost always contain fewer and safer excipients, the nonnutritional additives needed to manufacture tablets and capsules. For example, health food brands typically use cellulose (a plant compound) as a filler, whereas drugstore brands tend to use lactose (which is derived from dairy and is a common allergen).

Different companies sell variations on the multivitamin theme. There is no absolutely perfect formulation, only reasonable compro-mises. That's because it is physically impossible to get everything into one or two capsules or tablets, partly because some minerals are so bulky. Among the best multivitamin/mineral supplements are those made by Carlson, Solgar, and All One Nutritionals. Because combined multivitamin/multimineral supplements tend to scrimp on some miner-als—regardless of the brand—consider taking a separate multimineral supplement.

—m—

C-Reactive Protein: What You Need to Know

C-reactive protein, found in trace amounts in the blood of healthy people, has emerged as the leading marker of systemic (or bodywide) inflammation. People with elevated CRP levels are several times more likely to have a heart attack, compared with people who have normal levels of CRP, even if their cholesterol levels are normal. Furthermore, most serious degenerative diseases are also associated with high blood levels of CRP. If you are currently in good health but your CRP levels are elevated, health problems are quietly brewing.

It is easy and inexpensive to test your CRP, and you should ask your physician to measure your levels. Make sure, however, that your physician specifies the *high-sensitivity* (hs) or *ultra-sensitive* (us) CRP test. Older CRP tests are not very accurate.

- If your hsCRP level is less than 1 mg/L, you have a low risk of developing cardiovascular disease.
- If your hsCRP level is between 1 and 3 mg/L, you have an average risk of developing cardiovascular disease.
- If your hsCRP level is above 3 mg/L, you have a high risk of developing cardiovascular disease. Note: CRP levels can temporarily reach 400 to 500 mg/L in critically ill people.

CRP is not an absolutely perfect indicator of inflammation or predictor of disease risk. It is a sign of systemic inflammation, which may be related to cardiovascular disease, but it may also be symptomatic of other diseases, including cancer, inflammatory bowel disease, lupus, rheumatoid arthritis, and infection. If your CRP level is elevated, your physician should investigate other symptoms and risk factors. In addition, CRP levels may be normal in some people, but other markers of inflammation (such as sedimentation rate, myeloperoxidase, and different types of adhesion molecules) may be elevated. Few medical tests are definitive by themselves; they are most meaningful when viewed along with the results of other tests and symptoms.

— *m* —

Joseph: A Nonsurgical Treatment for Periodontal Disease

Sometimes people need a little nonnutritional help to eliminate an infection and control inflammation. That was the case with Joseph, whose dentist diagnosed him with a 9 mm pocket between two teeth—a space indicating a loss of bone and tissue and a sign of periodontal disease. His dentist referred him to a periodontist for surgery, which typically involves the painful removal of a small portion of gums. The theory is that healthier tissue will grow back.

But Joseph didn't relish the prospect of dental surgery—after all, who does?—so he investigated other approaches on the Internet. In the process, he discovered the dental research of Walter Loesche, D.M.D., Ph.D., a professor emeritus of the University of Michigan School of Dentistry, and Paul Keyes, D.D.S., of the National Institutes of Health. Both dentists have developed nonsurgical treatments for periodontal disease. The treatments involve "irrigating" under the gums with antibacterial compounds, including baking soda, salt, and commercial products such as Therasol. In this context, irrigation is simply a spray powered by a Via-Jet or WaterPik device. (See "Dental Inflammation" in chapter 12.)

Joseph, who lives in Phoenix, was able to locate William Helfert, D.D.S., in nearby Mesa, Arizona, who used these techniques to control pathogenic bacteria in the mouth. After an initial treatment in the office, Joseph continued the nightly five-minute treatments at home. A month later, his pocket was down to 5 mm, and after three months it was down to 3 mm. Joseph has continued the treatments at home, and his gums remain healthy. So far, he has not needed any dental surgery.

Some of the Benefits of a Multivitamin

Many of the nutrients in a multivitamin have direct or indirect anti-inflammatory benefits. Because nutrients work together as a biochemical team, their sum is usually greater than any of their individual contributions.

Vitamin A. In 1928, the *British Medical Journal* described vitamin A as the "anti-infective" vitamin. By protecting against infections, vitamin A reduces the likelihood of developing infection-related inflammation. Many supplements substitute beta-carotene for vitamin A, but the body's conversion of beta-carotene (found in carrots and other vegetables) is not always very efficient. The conversion depends on the health of your intestinal bacteria, whose activity may be reduced by poor diet, antibiotics, and acid-reducing drugs. Vitamin A is also needed for normal vision, and regular exposure to sunlight will increase vitamin A metabolism in the eyes and lead to a more rapid breakdown of the vitamin. Pregnant women or women who may become pregnant should not take more than 5,000 IU of vitamin A daily, but they can take more beta-carotene.

B-complex vitamins. Vitamins B_1, B_6, and B_{12}, especially when taken together (as they are in multivitamins and B-complex supplements), can significantly reduce musculoskeletal pain. Vitamin B_6 (100 to 200 mg daily) has been found to be helpful in treating carpal tunnel syndrome, although it will likely work better when combined with other B vitamins. A study of 303 elderly American military veterans found that chronic pain was strongly related to a deficiency of vitamin B_{12}, which affected 1 in 5 of the subjects. B-complex vitamins can also enhance the pain-relieving effects of nonsteroidal anti-inflammatory drugs (NSAIDs). The niacin form of vitamin B_3 (which causes a flush after you take it) reduces levels of C-reactive protein.

Vitamin C. Vitamin C is one of the most powerful scavengers of free radicals, and by quenching free radicals, vitamin C can dampen inflammatory reactions. In a study of 386 people, researchers found that C-reactive protein levels decreased by more than one-fourth after participants took 1,000 mg of vitamin C daily for two months. Vitamin C likely works through other mechanisms as well. For example, uncontrolled inflammation breaks down tissue. Because vitamin C is needed to make collagen, the most common protein in the body, it can strengthen tissue and may help the body resist inflammatory damage.

Vitamin D. In recent years, vitamin D has entered a nutrition renaissance. It helps strength both bones and muscles, reduces the risk of developing cancer and heart disease, and can even improve mood. In a study published in the *Archives of Internal Medicine* in 2008, researchers reported that daily supplements containing about 2,000 IU of vitamin D reduced nerve pain in people with type 2 diabetes. These analgesic benefits may extend to other conditions as well.

Vitamin D has long been known to improve and regulate immune function. Researchers recently discovered that vitamin D boosts levels of a highly specialized and powerful germ-killing peptide, cathelicidin, found in immune cells, skin, and other cells. Some researchers now believe that susceptibility to colds and flus is related to low wintertime levels of vitamin D. More than sixty studies have found that high levels of vitamin D reduce the risk of developing several cancers, including those of the breast, the colon, and the prostate. Another study reported that people taking vitamin D supplements were 8 percent less likely to die from *any* cause. Look for a multivitamin that provides 1,000 IU of vitamin D_3 daily. Otherwise, you may have to add a vitamin D supplement to bring your daily intake to between 1,000 and 2,000 IU daily.

Vitamin E. Although some recent studies have questioned vitamin E's benefits, the larger picture of scientific research still justifies supplement-ing with it. Vitamin E does reduce the risk of blood clots and heart disease, but, as with all other nutrients, it usually works best as part of a broader dietary and supplement regimen. In particular, several studies have found that natural-source vitamin E supplements can lower C-reactive protein levels by 30 to 50 percent. It has a variety of other anti-inflammatory benefits, such as turning off some of the genes involved in inflammation, reducing the activity of adhesion molecules, and being a mild Cox-2 inhibitor. Two studies have found that vitamin E supplements reduce pain in people with rheumatoid arthritis, although the effect is gradual. Other research found that a higher intake of vitamin E was associated with lower levels of immunoglobulin E (IgE), which is typically elevated in people with allergies.

Be sure that your supplement contains the natural form of vitamin E, which is identified as d-alpha tocopherol (or tocopheryl). It is assimilated twice as efficiently as the synthetic form, which is described as dl-alpha tocopherol in the fine print on labels. Although the alpha tocopherol form is the most biologically active, related compounds (such as gamma toco-pherol and tocotrienols) are also beneficial. Take 200 to 400 IU of vita-min E daily.

Vitamin K. It is difficult to find multivitamins that contain vitamin K, but hopefully this will soon change. Vitamin K is needed to make strong bones. The body uses vitamin K_1 to ensure normal clotting of the blood, whereas vitamin K_2 may help reduce the risk of coronary calcification (sometimes referred to as hardening of the arteries). Recent research indicates that vitamin K plays an important role in regulating blood sugar and may help prevent type 2 diabetes. That's significant because high blood sugar increases inflammation. Aim for 500 to 1,000 mcg of vita-min K daily. *Caution*: Vitamin K supplements may neutralize the effects of Coumadin and other blood thinners that inhibit vitamin K activity. If you take these drugs, check with your doctor first.

Calcium. Although calcium is usually thought of as a mineral that is needed for strong bones, it depends on vitamins D and K for normal uti-lization. It also teams up with magnesium in bones, as well as in regulat-ing heart rhythm. Considerable research indicates that calcium and vitamin D work together to maintain normal insulin function and glucose tolerance, which should help control inflammation.

Chromium. This mineral is probably more important than any other for the normal activity of insulin, a hormone that helps regulate blood sugar levels. Symptoms of chromium deficiency, including elevated blood glucose, insulin, total cholesterol, and triglycerides, can resemble those of prediabetes. This doesn't mean that a lack of chromium alone causes diabetes, but low chromium intake can contribute to diabetes. Chromium supplements may be of particular benefit in reducing weight, particularly among people who are depressed and overweight. Maintaining a normal weight is crucial for controlling inflammation because fat cells (particularly those around the belly) secrete two powerful promoters of inflammation, interleukin-6 and C-reactive protein. Take 500 mcg of either chromium polinicotinate (niacin bound) or chromium picolinate twice daily. The benefits will be enhanced when this supplement is combined with either a high-protein, low-carbohydrate diet or exercise.

Iodine. This mineral is needed to make the thyroid hormones thyroxine (T4) and triiodothyronine (T3). Many inflammatory symptoms may be caused by low thyroid gland activity, including arthritis and joint aches, allergies, asthma, muscular aches, itchiness, and hives. Several studies have found that large supplemental amounts of iodine can reduce viscous bronchial secretions in adults and children with asthma. The research suggests that iodine plays a role in modulating immune cells and may have anti-inflammatory benefits. Low thyroid (hypothyroidism) is underdiagnosed and often incorrectly treated when diagnosed. By middle age, many women have difficulty converting T4 to T3, the active form of the hormone. Physicians typically prescribe a synthetic form of T4, such as Levoxyl or Synthroid (levothyroxin). A better option is Armour thyroid hormone, a standardized natural product (porcine derived) that contains both T4 and T3. If you wish to avoid pork, consider asking your doctor for a prescription for Thyrolar, a synthetic combination of T4 and T3. Try taking 500 mcg to 4,000 mg of iodine daily, beginning at the lower dose.

Magnesium. Magnesium is the most versatile of all dietary minerals. It plays a role in more than three hundred chemical reactions, including in the production of nucleic acids and proteins, enzymes involved in making carbohydrates and fats, and the antioxidant glutathione. In the form of magnesium adenosine triphosphate (MgATP), magnesium provides energy for cells. Low magnesium levels can destabilize the energy-generating processes that occur in cells. When that happens, abnormally high levels of free radicals form, and they can damage tissues and stimulate inflammation. A recent cell study found that magnesium influences the rate of aging, with deficiencies accelerating the aging process. A lack of magnesium shortens telemeres, which are the tips of DNA sequences. Levels of inflammation typically increase with age, so slowing the aging process should help decrease inflammation.

Selenium. This mineral is a necessary part of several antioxidant enzymes called glutathione peroxidases. Glutathione peroxidases help prevent the formation of free radicals, and selenium also reduces the risk of cancer. In addition, selenium plays a role in the formation of thyroid hormones. (See iodine, on previous page.) Selenium supplements may be particularly beneficial for women who inherit mutations in the BRCA "cancer gene." Normally, this gene helps repair damaged genes, but the mutation increases the risk of developing breast and ovarian cancer. In a study of thirty-two women with BRCA gene mutations, researchers noted that they had a high rate of chromosome breaks, a cancer risk factor. After the women took selenium supplements for only three months, however, the rate of mutations decreased to that of normal women. Selenium also prevents mutations in the influenza (flu) virus and the coxsackie virus, which causes symptoms similar to those of the common cold. That's important because mutations in selenium-deficient people and animals result in much more dangerous viruses.

Zinc. Zinc plays many roles in helping to control inflammation. The body uses the mineral to make copper-zinc superoxide dismutase, a potent antioxidant, and a lack of zinc increases free radical activity. The body also uses zinc to make metallothionein, a protein that protects the body from toxic metals, such as lead and cadmium. Zinc can inhibit the replication of viruses, and zinc-containing Cold-Eeze lozenges can reduce cold symptoms and duration if taken on the first day of symptoms. Zinc works with copper, but the ratio between these two minerals is important. Excess zinc can impair immunity, so long-term use of supplemental zinc should be balanced with a small amount of copper. The amount of zinc should be fifteen to thirty times greater than that of copper.

Dr. Kunin and Susan: Antioxidants for Health

Years ago, Richard Kunin, M.D., of San Francisco, California, described himself as a "nasal neurotic." He had asthma, was allergic to dogs and cats, and sneezed literally a hundred times a day. He became interested in nutritional medicine, cured himself of all of his nasal and respiratory problems, and has gone on to become one of the most original thinkers in "orthomolecular medicine," which focuses on using nutrition to achieve optimal health.

More recently, Kunin has been investigating the relationship between nutrition, blood coagulation, and health. All of this relates to inflammation because low blood flow (ischemia) generates excessive free radicals, which activate inflammation-promoting cytokines that in turn increase blood clotting and alter normal heart rhythms.

One patient, Susan, had high blood pressure much of her adult life but chose not to treat it medically. By her late sixties, she had undergone a triple coronary-artery bypass. She consulted Kunin after repeated attacks of angina (heart pain), arrhythmias after exercising, muscle aches, postoperative memory loss, bronchitis, and coughing. Memory loss is common after bypass surgery, and Susan had difficulty recalling her recent medical history.

Based on Susan's medical history and laboratory tests, Kunin diagnosed her high prothrombin (blood clotting) activity and felt that it was likely the result of a genetic propensity toward excessive blood clotting. He also felt that Susan's muscle aches were caused by the statin drug interfering with her body's production of vitaminlike coenzyme Q_{10}.

Susan had an acute sense of smell, which Kunin recognized as a probable sign of chemical sensitivity. The most likely culprit was Susan's forced-air gas furnace. Such furnaces, as well as gas stoves, release burned hydrocarbons into the air, and sensitive people react to these compounds. Kunin recommended that she replace the filter and update her heating system.

Kunin then developed an antioxidant and anticoagulant regimen for Susan to follow, based in part on the fact that vitamin antioxidants also have blood-thinning properties. Bromelain supplements served as a natural way to reduce blood viscosity (caused by excessive fibrin), as did small oral amounts of heparin, an anticoagulant drug. Heparin, Kunin explained, has anticoagulant effects when taken orally (not only by injection) but does not interfere with vitamin K metabolism the way that Coumadin does. Kunin also recommended that she take supplements of the herb *Ginkgo biloba*, which reduces the risk of blood clots. Among the other supplements she took were B vitamins, vitamin C, vitamin E, alpha-lipoic acid, and the amino acid L-arginine.

Susan's health has improved considerably. Her blood pressure has been lowered, and she no longer has arrhythmias or muscle aches.

Recommended Multivitamin Supplements

It is very important to take a high-potency multivitamin and multimineral supplement. I recommend three specific multivitamins. Because nearly all multivitamins tend to be low in minerals, please consider adding a separate multimineral supplement.

1. *Carlson Multi-Gel.* This is one of the few high-potency multivitamin supplements that also contains adequate levels of minerals. In all, it provides thirteen vitamins and seventeen minerals in three daily capsules. Multi-Gel has 1,000 mg of calcium and 400 mg of magnesium, two important minerals that often get shortchanged in other supplements. (For more information, visit carlsonlabs.com or call 800-323-4141.)

2. *Carlson Nutra-Support Diabetes.* This supplement provides 20 mg of the main B-complex vitamins, along with several ingredients (such as alpha-lipoic acid and silymarin) geared toward maintaining normal blood sugar. It is one of the few multivitamins that includes ample amounts of vitamin K_2. This supplement does not contain iron, which is good because excess iron is associated with inflammation and a higher risk of developing heart disease. (For more information, visit carlsonlabs.com.)

3. *Solgar VM-Prime.* VM-75 Vegetable Capsules. This is a very high-potency multivitamin supplement. An iron-free version is available in tablet form. (For more information, visit solgar.com.)

4. *All One Nutritionals.* Some people do not like taking capsules and tablets, and All One Multiple Vitamins and Minerals Powder is an acceptable product. It is designed to be mixed in a glass of juice or water. Note that it is sweetened with maltodextrin, a type of sugar. (For more information, visit all–one.com.)

In the next chapter I focus on glucosamine, chondroitin, and other supplements helpful in treating osteoarthritis and in maintaining healthy cartilage throughout the body. The reason is that osteoarthritis is an all-too-common and debilitating health problem, and these supplements are among the most widely used anti-inflammatory products on the market.

CHAPTER 11

Glucosamine, Chondroitin, and Other Supplements for Osteoarthritis

Glucosamine and chondroitin are among the most popular of all dietary supplements, and they are most often used to reduce the pain and inflammation associated with osteoarthritis. A sizable body of human research supports the benefits of these two supplements. Recently, however, a couple of highly publicized studies have raised some doubts about their benefits. Although it can be difficult to navigate through the science, only one conclusion can be drawn from all of the evidence: these supplements do reduce pain and inflammation related to osteoarthritis of the knees, and some research shows that glucosamine can even regenerate worn or damaged joint cartilage.

This chapter describes some of the compelling research on glucosamine and chondroitin, as well as a few of the confusing and controversial studies. I will also discuss several other nutrients that help in treating osteoarthritis. For example, vitamin C works with glucosamine and chondroitin to make cartilage. In addition, supplemental methylsulfonylmethane (MSM), S-adenosylmethionine (SAMe), rose hips, and denatured type 2 cartilage may help reduce pain. Pycnogenol and 5-Loxin are also helpful, and although I have already discussed these two supplements, I will return to them briefly.

Why devote an entire chapter to osteoarthritis, when this and many other inflammatory conditions will be discussed in the next chapter? There are two reasons. One is the sheer popularity of glucosamine and chondroitin supplements, and the other is that these (and the other supplements) appear to have health benefits far beyond their roles in lessening the symptoms of osteoarthritis.

The Basics of Cartilage

Your body consists of a biological matrix that is dependent on proteins, fats, minerals, and vitamins. Cartilage is one of the principal soft structural materials of the body. Your nose, ears, tendons, and ligaments are made of cartilage.

The exact composition of cartilage varies somewhat, depending on its location and function in the body. The cartilage forming the pads in your joints, such as your knees, is denser than other types of cartilage. These pads are known as "articular cartilage" because they are located where the body articulates, or moves. Articular cartilage in the knees absorbs the physical impact of walking, thus keeping the interlocking bones of joints from grinding against one another. This type of cartilage, along with related chemical compounds in the elbows, the fingers, and the mandibular joints of the jaw, also provides a smooth surface that enables the joints to swivel. When articular cartilage wears out, the nearby bones rub against one another, leading to excessive wear and tear, inflammation, and pain.

The best way to think about glucosamine, chondroitin, and other "cartilage nutrients" is as the bricks and mortar and the lubricating fluid of joints. Specialized cells called chondrocytes make cartilage. Cartilage is 80 percent water, which helps reduce friction and allows it to bounce back after being compressed. Two types of protein—collagen proteins and noncollagen proteins—make up most of the remainder of cartilage. (Collagen, by the way, is the predominant protein in the body.)

The building blocks of all protein in our bodies comes from the food we eat. Approximately 90 to 98 percent of the collagen protein consists of "collagen type 2," and the remainder is collagen types 5, 6, 9, 10, and

11. The differences among these collagens are based on slight variations of protein structure. Vitamin C is needed to make all forms of collagen.

Meanwhile, the noncollagen proteins consist primarily of proteoglycans, a type of protein-sugar molecule. Aggrecan is the chief type of proteoglycan, but all types of proteoglycans consist of several glycosaminoglycans. These glycosaminoglycans include chondroitin sulfate, hyaluronic acid, keratan sulfate 1, and heparin sulfate, among others. Glucosamine sulfate is necessary to make glycosaminoglycans.

You can see from this brief discussion that glucosamine and chondroitin are essential constituents of articular cartilage, but there are several other interesting aspects to cartilage structure. First, articular cartilage consists of four distinct layers. The softest layer is farthest from the bone, and the amount of mineralization (calcium, phosphorus, and magnesium) increases closer to the bone, which forms the fourth layer. Second, several enzymes, including collagenase, aggrecanase, and hyaluronidase, break down cartilage. Normally, these enzymes are part of the process of removing damaged or old cells. But when the body tips toward a chronic inflammatory state, the activity of these enzymes increases, leading to an accelerated breakdown of cartilage and to pain and stiffness.

I wrote in chapter 5 that common analgesic drugs, such as ibuprofen, aspirin, and acetaminophen, hasten the breakdown of cartilage. The occasional use of these drugs should not pose a problem, but taking them on a regular basis also increases the risk of gastric ulcers, heart attack, and heart failure. The irony is all too obvious: people take these drugs to ease their osteoarthritic pain, and although the drugs do in fact reduce pain, they speed the underlying disease process.

The Research on Glucosamine and Chondroitin

More than forty studies with people support the benefits of glucosamine and chondroitin in reducing the pain and stiffness of arthritis or in increasing the thickness of cartilage pads. Even the so-called negative studies show clear benefits.

Some of the studies have been small, and others have included large numbers of people. In an eight-week study, researchers gave glucosamine, chondroitin, and magnesium ascorbate (a form of vitamin C) supplements to thirty-two Navy SEALs who had either chronic knee or lower-back pain. The supplements lessened knee pain by 26 to 43 percent but did not help with back pain. In a separate study, doctors used similar supplements to treat ninety-three patients with osteoarthritis of the knees. Fifty-two percent of the patients had a more than 25 percent reduction in symptoms, twice the number of those who improved after taking placebos.

In two studies, Jean-Yves Reginster, M.D., Ph.D., of the University of Liege, Belgium, used digital X-rays to precisely measure knee cartilage in 106 patients with osteoarthritis. After taking glucosamine supplements (1,500 mg daily) for three years, most patients had no loss of cartilage and many had improvements, along with significant reductions in pain. Meanwhile, those who took placebos lost cartilage. In a follow-up analysis of fifteen human studies, Reginster noted that glucosamine increased joint cartilage, reduced the noncartilage space in knee joints, lessened pain, and improved mobility.

Even people who took and later stopped taking glucosamine supplements benefited over the long term. Olivier Bruyere, Ph.D., of the University of Liege, Belgium, and his colleagues tracked 272 patients from two earlier studies in which the subjects took either 1,500 mg of glucosamine sulfate or placebos daily for one to three years. The patients stopped taking the supplements (or placebos) after the trials. Five years later, Bruyere followed up and found that patients who had taken glucosamine sulfate were 57 percent less likely to have undergone total joint-replacement surgery, according to a report in *Osteoarthritis and Cartilage*. In contrast, people who had taken placebos were more than twice as likely to undergo this type of surgery.

The Controversial GAIT Study

The Glucosamine/Chondroitin Arthritis Intervention Trial (GAIT), which initially included 1,583 patients with osteoarthritis, has turned out to be one of the most controversial studies involving these supplements. Several medical journal articles and scores of newspaper reports emphasized that glucosamine and chondroitin had no benefits in treating osteoarthritis. Yet it often seemed as if few people had read the actual GAIT results, which tended to be positive. Confused? I'll clarify the findings.

On November 14, 2005, the initial results of the GAIT study were presented at a meeting of the American College of Rheumatology in San Diego, California. The subjects took the following supplements or medications daily: 1,500 mg of glucosamine hydrochloride; 1,200 mg of chondroitin sulfate; both supplements; the drug Celebrex; or placebos. The study was "double blind," in that neither the patients nor their doctors were aware of what they were taking. Overall, neither the supplements nor the drug led to any reduction in pain. In patients with moderate to severe knee pain, however—those most likely to require intervention in the real world—78 percent responded significantly to the combination of glucosamine and chondroitin. The combination of these two supplements was significantly better than either supplement by itself or Celebrex. People with mild osteoarthritic pain did not seem to benefit, but it's difficult to discern improvements or setbacks in patients who have mild knee pain.

In 2008, the researchers reported the results of 572 patients who had been tracked for two years. Based on X-ray evidence, the researchers concluded that the loss of joint cartilage in any of the treatment groups was not significantly different from that of the placebo group. But the study had numerous flaws that went largely unreported, although the researchers did acknowledge problems with their data in their scientific report in the journal *Arthritis & Rheumatism*. For example, the progression of osteoarthritis among people taking placebos was less than half of what had been anticipated, which would have invalidated any comparisons. Several other problems plagued the study. One, the number of patients was too small and, two, the study's duration was too short, which limited the statistical findings of the study. (A minimum of three years' treatment is needed to ascertain benefits.) Three, the X-ray instrumentation was not sensitive enough to make clinically meaningful measurements.

That said, the researchers found that glucosamine hydrochloride supplements did yield better results than placebos or any of the other treatments. In effect, patients taking glucosamine supplements had a slight increase in joint cartilage—a benefit that was about eight and one-half times greater than among people taking Celebrex. Inexplicably, though, people taking a combination of glucosamine and chondroitin experienced the greatest progression of joint damage, a finding that (given all of the research on the subject) just didn't make sense.

Does the Form of Glucosamine Make a Difference?

Glucosamine supplements are sold in two forms: glucosamine sulfate and glucosamine hydrochloride. In an analysis of human studies using the different forms, researchers noted that most of the negative studies on glucosamine had used the hydrochloride form. In contrast, most of the positive trials were performed with glucosamine sulfate. The researchers concluded that the sulfate part of the molecule (consisting of one sulfur and four oxygen molecules) may contribute to the benefits of glucosamine in osteoarthritis.

Sulfate, a form of the mineral sulfur, is virtually ignored as a nutrient, yet it is an essential constituent of tissue. Sulfur compounds occur in many amino acids, vitamin B_1, biotin, glutathione, alpha-lipoic acid, and coenzyme A, which drive cellular energy production. The mineral is found in most of the supplements that are used to treat osteoarthritis, such as glucosamine sulfate, chondroitin sulfate, methylsulfonylmethane, and N-adenosylmethionine. Sulfur also has a role in fortifying the tissues that form skin, hair, nails, and cartilage.

There is additional evidence that sulfate (i.e., a sulfur-oxygen molecule) is more important than glucosamine, per se. In a small but noteworthy study, John L. Hoffer, M.D., Ph.D., of McGill University in Montreal, reported that glucosamine supplements do not increase blood levels of glucosamine. The synthesis of glycosaminoglycans, however, does depend on blood sulfate levels, and Hoffer found that both blood and joint levels of sulfate increased 13 percent within hours of a person taking a glucosamine sulfate supplement. The study also found that sulfate levels decreased 11 percent when acetaminophen was given with 1 gram of glucosamine sulfate. This study points to the value of sulfate, as well as to the potential damage to cartilage from a common analgesic drug.

Glucosamine hydrochloride does benefit some people, and it seems to work reasonably well when combined with chondroitin, which provides sulfate. It is very possible that the effectiveness of glucosamine hydrochloride depends on the amount of sulfur in the diet or on other supplements. Eggs and cruciferous vegetables are very high in sulfur, as are many supplements (which will be discussed shortly). But as far as supplements go, glucosamine sulfate does seem to be the more bioactive form.

Does Glucosamine Negatively Affect Blood Sugar?

In 1999, a letter to the journal *Lancet* raised questions about whether glucosamine supplements would increase blood sugar, cause insulin resistance, and lead to or aggravate type 2 diabetes. The questions raised in this letter were widely reported in health newsletters, which turned the letter about glucosamine into a warning. The issue has since become the stuff of urban legends—untrue.

As the *University of California Berkeley Wellness Letter* and the *Tufts University Health & Nutrition Letter* were mailing their warnings to subscribers, the *Lancet* published several new letters that balanced the brewing controversy. These follow-up letters noted that the original one was highly speculative and based only on limited animal research. In contrast, clinical experiences with people indicated that glucosamine supplements might actually lead to a slight lowering of blood sugar levels. One researcher pointed out that glucosamine supplements improved wound healing (an indication of their tissue-supporting role beyond that of joints), reduced headaches, and eased inflammatory bowel disease in patients. The positive letters in the *Lancet* were ignored by the Berkeley and Tufts newsletters, as well as by newspapers and magazines. A more recent study, published in 2007 in *Diabetes Care*, confirmed the safety of glucosamine. Supplements did not affect either blood sugar levels or cholesterol.

How to Take Glucosamine and Chondroitin

One of the foremost experts on osteoarthritis and the author of *The Arthritis Cure*, Jason Theodosakis, M.D., told me that most patients with osteoarthritis can reduce their medication dosages and completely stop taking pain-killing drugs after six to nine months of supplementation. He recommends that patients with osteoarthritis—or those at risk, such as from years of jogging—take 1,500 mg of glucosamine and 1,200 mg of chondroitin daily. This is the effective dose in most studies. Do note that glucosamine is extracted from the shells of crustaceans, so you should not take it if you have allergies to shellfish. Chondroitin is extracted from the tracheas of cows.

Other Supplements That Help with Osteoarthritis

Several other supplements also help in reducing the inflammation, pain, and swelling of osteoarthritis. Many of the supplements that are beneficial in osteoarthritis contain sulfur. These supplements include glucosamine sulfate, chondroitin sulfate, methylsulfonylmethane, and S-adenosylmethionine.

Vitamin C. This essential nutrient is required to make collagen, one of the proteins that forms cartilage. Many glucosamine and chondroitin supplements contain some vitamin C, but most adults likely need at least 1 gram daily.

Methylsulfonylmethane (*MSM*). MSM is chemically related to dimethyl sulfoxide (DMSO), which has a long history of use as a topical analgesic in veterinary and alternative medicine. MSM is the oral form and has been found to reduce pain in people with osteoarthritis. One study reported significant improvements with 3 grams of MSM taken daily for twelve weeks. Taking 1,500 mg of MSM in combination with glucosamine sulfate was especially beneficial.

Avocado/soybean unsaponifiables (*ASU*). The odd name refers to particular fatty extracts of the avocado and the soybean. ASU has been found to reduce pain, slow the breakdown of existing cartilage, and stimulate the production of new cartilage. It works in part by reducing the activity of inflammatory cytokines. An article in *Osteoarthritis and Cartilage* reviewed four published studies of ASU in people and found that supplements reduced pain in people with knee osteoarthritis.

S-adenosyl-L-methionine (*SAMe*). Pronounced "sammy," this sulfur-containing nutrient contributes to hundreds of chemical reactions in the body. Methyl groups provide carbon and hydrogen and are necessary for creating new cells. SAMe has often been recommended for treating inflammation and arthritis: it likely donates sulfur molecules to glucosamine and chondroitin sulfate, enabling the body to build new collagen and cartilage.

Rose hips. This is the ripe red fruit of roses, most often seen on wild roses in autumn. Popular in the 1970s, rose hips have largely receded in the supplement marketplace. A meta-analysis of three studies, published in *Osteoarthritis and Cartilage* in 2008, found that taking 5 grams daily of rose hips led to a substantial decrease in pain (twice that of the placebo groups) in more than three hundred patients with osteoarthritis.

5-Loxin. This standardized, proprietary extract of *Boswellia serrata* can significantly reduce symptoms of knee osteoarthritis, according to a study by U.S. and Indian researchers.

Pycnogenol. This extract of French maritime pine bark can reduce pain and inflammation caused by osteoarthritis. It's supported by several human studies.

Type 2 collagen. More than 90 percent of the collagen in cartilage consists of type 2 collagen. In recent years, numerous studies have found that type 2 collagen, obtained from chicken or bovine sources, stimulates the synthesis of chondrocytes. A small study of people found that taking supplements of cartilage type 2 did result in less pain and greater mobility in patients; however, the benefits of type 2 cartilage appear greater in patients with rheumatoid arthritis. I recommend the *un*denatured type 2 cartilage.

PART IV

Putting Anti-Inflammation Syndrome Nutrients to Work for You

CHAPTER 12

The Inflammation Syndrome, Diseases, and Specific Conditions

Up to this point we have focused on the dietary causes and solutions for the inflammation syndrome. In this chapter we shift to specific diseases and conditions that are caused or exacerbated by inflammation—and are remedied by improvements in diet and by taking anti-inflammatory supplements.

Inflammatory disorders frequently follow a progression beginning with mild symptoms that, if the underlying causes remain uncorrected, lead to more serious and difficult-to-treat diseases. For example, gastritis can lead to stomach ulcers and increase the risk of developing stomach cancer. Similarly, athletic injuries can set the stage for osteoarthritis and chronic musculoskeletal pain. Although symptoms may seem to be mild or transitory during the early stages of an inflammatory disease, it is easier to permanently heal them at this time. In contrast, it is more difficult to reverse established diseases because of the extent of tissue damage.

In addition, inflammatory disorders often occur in clusters, one disorder being linked to another and often forming the inflammation syndrome. These clusters point to common underlying causes, although the causes may be overlooked. For example, periodontitis increases the risk of developing heart disease, making some physicians believe that both

177

diseases have a common infectious cause. Rather, people with the two conditions are more likely to share a common inflammatory pattern resulting from a pro-inflammatory diet. As another example, people with asthma frequently suffer from depression. The depression does not result from the diagnosis of asthma but instead may be symptomatic of the same fatty-acid imbalance affecting body and mind.

You might wonder why, if most people have essentially the same pro-inflammatory diet, one person develops a particular set of symptoms, such as rheumatoid arthritis, whereas another suffers asthmatic attacks, and yet another person has heart disease. The diseases to which you are susceptible reflect your individual biological weaknesses, which are the result of your genetics, overall lifestyle, stresses, age, and diet. To understand this, it helps to see your genes and biochemistry as a series of chainlike links. Everyone has his or her own set of weak links (as well as strong links), and the number of weak links increases with age, poor diet, stress, and other insults. Your major weak links may be your heart, your joints, or your stomach or some other tissue. Good nutrition reinforces these links and may be more important to health than is genetics; this has been borne out by recent research. As you read earlier in this book, genes themselves depend on the body receiving adequate levels of nutrients for optimal functioning.

In general, the following sections place more emphasis on conditions affecting larger numbers of people and less emphasis on those affecting fewer people. It would be impossible to cover the full spectrum of inflammatory diseases in this type of book. Still, the AI Diet Plan should have a positive affect on virtually all inflammatory diseases. So if you suffer from a disorder that is not described here, it would be worthwhile for you to try the diet plan and some of the supplements.

Age-Related Wear and Tear

What Is Age-Related Wear and Tear?

Throughout a person's life, old or damaged cells are broken down and replaced. After about age twenty-seven, however, the rate of cell damage begins to outpace the body's natural repair processes. With poor nutrition, this shift toward greater cellular breakdown may begin at an earlier age. Old cells are not as efficient as new ones, and the accumulation of old cells is what is recognized as aging.

Causes

Wear and tear is a normal part of living and aging. Much of it results from damage by free radicals, according to Denham Harman, M.D., Ph.D., a professor emeritus at the University of Nebraska, Omaha. In the 1950s, Harman proposed the free-radical theory of aging, stating that these hazardous molecules chip away at the deoxyribonucleic acid (DNA), the proteins, and the fats in cells. The cumulative effect is less efficient cell performance and decreased activity of organs, reflected in a weaker heart and weaker lungs, as but two examples. Sometimes free-radical mutations of DNA lead to vastly different cell behavior, such as that of cancer cells.

Most of these free radicals are generated by normal metabolic processes in the body, such as the burning of glucose for energy or the detoxification of dangerous chemicals, such as cigarette smoke. Normally, most of these free radicals are contained in specific chemical reactions, but some do leak out—and additional free radicals may be formed when a person consumes inadequate levels of antioxidants.

Some people seem to age faster than others, a process strongly linked to excessive levels of free radicals. A good example is a woman who maintains a beautiful tan in her twenties and thirties, either by sunning herself on the beach or by using tanning booths. By the time she turns fifty, she will likely have far more facial wrinkles and tougher skin than a person who has minimized his or her exposure to the sun. That's because tanning increases exposure to ultraviolet radiation, which creates free radicals and speeds the aging of skin cells. Athletic injuries can also accelerate the aging process, particularly of joints and bones, and injuries have been documented to create free radicals. The chemicals in cigarette smoke are dangerous in part because they stress the body's ability to detoxify them, generating still more free radicals in the process.

In addition, poor nutrition and leading a hard life increase wear and tear. For example, malnourished people often look ten to fifteen years older than their chronological age. Good nutrition should provide compounds that maintain a normal aging process or, ideally, even slow it down. Inadequate nutrition hurts our natural defenses against a variety of stresses, such as UV radiation, air pollution, and noxious chemicals.

How Common Is Age-Related Wear and Tear?

The sad fact is that everyone ages, and everyone will experience some degree of age-related wear and tear, even while remaining in "good health" late in life. Frailty late in life is one sign of wear and tear.

The Inflammation Syndrome Connection

Much of the cleanup of old cells is performed by the immune system, chiefly various types of white blood cells. Increased wear and tear activates more white blood cells, which are a double-edged sword because they secrete more inflammation-producing chemicals. Immune cells may target specific sites in the body, such as joints, the heart, or the bronchi, or may migrate and cause more systemic inflammation. A study in the *Archives of Internal Medicine* described a strong relationship between frailty in elderly men and women and high levels of C-reactive protein and other signs of chronic inflammation. In addition, frail elderly people also had elevated prediabetic levels of glucose and insulin. All of these factors contribute to the breakdown and aging of tissues—that is, age-related wear and tear—which evolves into a wasting syndrome among many elderly people.

Standard Treatment

There is really no treatment for the normal process of aging, although some hormones may restore many aspects of youthfulness, such as muscle and sexual vigor. Certain medications may also improve cognitive function, but nearly all drugs possess undesirable side effects. For example, many hormones can increase cancer risk.

Nutrients That Can Help

Antioxidants such as vitamins E, C, and others often have been described as "antiaging" nutrients because they quench many of the excess free radicals. Consuming a lot of vegetables and fruits and taking antioxidant supplements strengthen the body's defenses against free radicals. Antioxidants also have potent anti-inflammatory properties.

The most significant recent research has focused on resveratrol, a plant extract that activates Sirt1, a gene that regulates longevity. Researchers who conducted animal studies have found that supplemental resveratrol increases longevity. The limited human research has shown that resveratrol improves blood sugar levels in people with type 2 diabetes, a change that should positively affect aging. Other supplements (such as chromium) that regulate blood sugar should also slow the aging process.

What Else Might Help?

High levels of two hormones, insulin and cortisol, appear to speed the aging process. Insulin is usually regarded as the hormone needed to burn blood sugar, but elevated insulin levels speed up the aging process and increase the risk of developing coronary artery disease. A diet relatively low in refined sugars and carbohydrates, such as the diet described in this book, can help blood sugar and insulin levels, which in turn will decrease inflammation levels.

Cortisol is one of the body's primary stress-response hormones, and high levels stress the body itself, leading to wear and tear. Cortisol also increases a person's risk of having a heart attack. The body cannot maintain a biological red alert without paying the price. Stress-reduction techniques, as well as the B-complex vitamins, can lower cortisol levels. See the section on Diabetes.

Allergies, Food

What Are Food Allergies?

Various types of food allergies or food sensitivities (characterized by symptoms, but not confirmed by laboratory tests) can maintain the body's inflammatory response at a high idle. These allergies can exacerbate symptoms of other inflammatory diseases, such as asthma and rheumatoid arthritis, or raise blood pressure and blood sugar levels. Occasionally, they can completely mimic the symptoms of other diseases.

Causes

There are several leading causes of food allergies, and they may intertwine. Physicians have traditionally recognized only acute allergic reactions, such as when a person develops a rash after eating shellfish or strawberries. Most cases of food allergies, however, may be more subtle and difficult to diagnose.

Food Addictions

As ironic as it might seem, some people actually become addicted to a food that causes an allergic reaction. This allergy/addiction may develop as part of the body's response to a commonly consumed allergen. During these reactions, the body releases endorphins, substances that create a natural "high." Any substance that creates a temporary sense of euphoria can become addictive, and in this case people can develop an addiction to the allergenic food, initiating the high.

Often, eating a lot of any particular food (even healthy foods) can create an allergy to it because, inexplicably, it triggers an immune response or it stresses specific digestive enzymes. It is as if too much of any single type of food overloads the body's ability to continue to break it down in the gut. Furthermore, any food can be the source of an allergy/addiction, whether it is junk food or a healthy food. One clue to an allergy/addiction is a food that a person craves. Foods containing chocolate, dairy, wheat, corn, tomatoes, and soy are among the most common food allergens.

Celiac Disease

Wheat, rye, and barley contain *gluten*, a term used to describe a family of about forty proteins. (Note: Amaranth, buckwheat, corn, millet, rice, sorghum, and soy flours are gluten free. Oats do not contain gluten, but they are often contaminated with it. Pure buckwheat is not a grain, but it may be blended with refined or whole wheat.) People who are gluten-sensitive often develop celiac disease, but nonceliac gluten sensitivity may be common. The immune response to gluten can damage the wall of the intestine, resulting in explosive bowel movements, poor nutrient absorption, and a consequential increased risk of contracting dozens of diseases. Celiac disease can also trigger immune responses without any gastrointestinal symptoms. For example, British researchers reported in the journal *Neurology* that gluten sensitivity was the cause of headaches and the likely cause of inflamed brain tissue. Another study, published in the October 2001 *Rheumatology*, reported that 40 percent of subjects who began to follow a gluten-free diet had a reduction in rheumatoid arthritis symptoms.

Specifically, celiac disease significantly increases the risk of getting a skin condition known as dermatitis herpetiformus, gastroesophageal reflux disorder (GERD), iron-deficiency anemia, irritable bowel syndrome, lactose intolerance, osteoporosis, and thyroid disease.

Leaky Gut Syndrome

Leaky gut refers to an abnormal permeability of the stomach and intestine wall, allowing incompletely digested proteins to enter the bloodstream. When such proteins move into the bloodstream, they trigger an immune response. Leaky gut is common in people with celiac disease, and it also may increase the likelihood of a variety of nongluten-related food allergies. A leaky gut can be caused by nutritional deficiencies, stress, stomach flu, antibiotics, and just about anything else that irritates the gut wall.

Nightshade Sensitivity

Some people, including an estimated 20 percent of people with rheumatoid arthritis, react to one or all nightshade foods, which include tomatoes, potatoes, eggplant, peppers, tomatillos, and tobacco (that is chewed or smoked rather than eaten). The reaction may be allergic in nature, or it may be that some people are very sensitive to small amounts of toxins in these foods.

How Common Are Food Allergies?

No one has precise numbers of the prevalence of food allergies and allergy-like sensitivities. Conventional allergists will often say they are rare, whereas physicians who routinely treat them may claim that 90 percent of people have at least one food allergy. The numbers of people with celiac disease are more precise, with the disease affecting about 1 in every 111 people—approximately 3 million Americans and 1 percent of the world population. Nonceliac gluten sensitivity, with often subtle symptoms, may affect half of the population, according to some estimates.

The Inflammation Syndrome Connection

Food allergies with a documented elevation of IgE and IgA antibodies reflect an immune system that has been unnecessarily stirred up; however, not all food allergies trigger these specific immune responses. It is possible that other types of immune reactions will eventually be identified or that a person's symptoms occur through some other mechanism.

Allergic reactions may be greatest in one part of the body, such as in the gut or the nasal area, but activated immune cells migrate throughout the body and frequently attack healthy cells, causing a wide variety of symptoms. In a sense, an allergic reaction shifts the normal biochemistry to a status resembling a military yellow or red alert. Such a heightened state boosts levels of other substances, such as adrenaline and the stress hormone cortisol. All of these stressful changes take a toll on the body and help deplete nutrients, so it is wise to reduce the symptoms of food allergies to relieve immediate discomfort and to lessen long-term wear and tear.

Standard Treatment

Conventional treatment of food allergens, when they are recognized, consists of avoidance.

Dietary Changes and Nutrients That Can Help

It is best to avoid foods that trigger allergic reactions. In addition, a rotation diet, in which the same food families are eaten only once every four days, may reduce the chances of future allergies developing. Avoiding an allergenic food for six months to a year sometimes allows the immune system to recover and not react to the problem food, as long as it is not consumed too often.

Several studies have found that a low intake of fish and fish oils or a high intake of refined oils (such as margarine) is associated with a wide range of allergylike symptoms, rheumatoid arthritis, and asthma. Eating more fish and taking omega-3 fish oil supplements are likely to help, assuming that you are not allergic to the fish.

Sometimes concomitant allergies magnify a reaction. Concomitant allergies are a little like binary weapons, with both parts being relatively innocuous until they are combined. Corn and banana, egg and apple, pork and black pepper, and milk and chocolate are common concomitant allergens. So are a variety of pollens and foods, such as ragweed and egg or milk, juniper and beef, and elm and milk.

What Else Might Help?

Because damage to the gut wall is often involved in food allergies, several supplements might be useful in healing the digestive tract. Glutamine, an amino acid, plays an important role in gut-wall integrity. *Probiotics*, the term used to describe supplements of "good" gut bacteria, might also be helpful. Various digestive aid supplements, containing pancreatic or plant enzymes, might promote the complete digestion of food. Serenaid, a supplement that breaks down gluten, might help people deal with small and occasional amounts of gluten in the diet; it is available from Klaire Laboratories (888-488-2488).

When it is not possible to avoid a food, "neutralization" therapy might help. Minute amounts of an extract of an allergenic food are held under the tongue, from where they rapidly enter the bloodstream. It appears that the right dosage can inhibit the body's response to the allergen. The dosage has to be determined through *provocation* testing, which is done by a type of allergist known as a *clinical ecologist*.

Yeast (*Candida albicans*) infections can sometimes be the hidden source of many food allergies. People are most likely to develop a yeast infection after undergoing antibiotic therapy, which kills both good and bad bacteria in the gut. *Candida* is an opportunistic infection, and doctors often overlook it. When the yeast infection is successfully treated (with a combination of prescription antifungal medications and over-the-counter probiotics), food allergies may disappear.

Allergies, Inhalant

What Are Inhalant Allergies?

Inhalant allergies are immune system overreactions (hypersensitivities) to any type of otherwise innocuous substances, such as pollens, molds, and cat dander. These types of allergies typically elevate blood levels of immunoglobulin E (IgE), which is part of the immune response. Pollen allergies tend to be seasonal, causing reactions only when a specific grass or tree blooms, although some people react to many different pollens throughout much of the year. The most common symptom is rhinitis, which, in practical terms, means nasal inflammation, an itchy and runny nose, sneezing, and nasal congestion.

The term *atopic disease* is often used to describe inhalant allergies, but it is often inappropriate. Atopic suggests that such allergies are inherited. While people with allergies are likely to have allergic children, it is now common for children to develop pollen allergies even though their parents and grandparents never experienced them.

Causes

Whenever an immune system reacts to something, such as ragweed pollen, when it shouldn't, it is obvious that something serious has gone awry. Pollens or dander are misidentified by immune cells as threats, triggering a massive and physically uncomfortable response. While medical and drug researchers are trying to figure out the molecular details of what goes wrong, they miss the obvious: allergies, on the scale that they now exist, are a recent phenomenon. So what has changed?

Research conducted by Francis Pottenger, M.D., during the 1930s offers a clue about how modern dietary changes have led to significant increases in the prevalence of allergies. Pottenger conducted a variety of dietary studies on more than nine hundred cats. He found that when the quality of their diets declined, health problems developed and grew worse with each subsequent generation that had the same poor diet. By the third generation, 90 percent of the cats with poor diets had developed allergies and skin diseases (which were usually manifestations of allergy). Many vitamins and minerals are needed for normal functioning of the immune system, and suboptimal levels of nutrients and deficiencies impair the normal programming of immunity.

Pottenger found that this trend could be reversed in the second generation, but that it took four generations of normal feeding to once again yield healthy nonallergic cats. That reversal was not possible by the third generation of cats that had a nutritionally deficient diet. Furthermore, the cats became incapable of reproducing by the fourth generation, the last.

If you see parallels between the lives of Pottenger's cats and people today, you are on the right track. Based on the prevalence of allergies, many people (and families) are in the equivalent of second and third generations having poor diets; one of every five American couples is infertile.

How Common Are Inhalant Allergies?

Inhalant allergies have become very common in Western industrialized nations but are rare in less developed countries. Approximately 20 percent of Americans have allergies, which translates to almost 60 million people. As many as 17 million Americans also have nonallergic rhinitis, and 22 million have a combination of allergic and nonallergic rhinitis. Nonallergic rhinitis refers to the symptoms but without any identifiable allergic cause. According to Robert S. Ivker, D.O., of Denver, Colorado, 40 million Americans suffer from sinusitis, one manifestation of rhinitis. Given all of the manifestations of allergies, their prevalence (diagnosed and undiagnosed) is likely in the neighborhood of 100 million.

The Inflammation Syndrome Connection

The first phase of allergic rhinitis involves sneezing and a runny nose after exposure to an allergen. This is followed by an increase in eosinophils, immune cells that promote inflammation, and, equally important, set the stage for a hair-trigger immune response after further exposures to the allergen.

Researchers believe that a shift in the ratio between two types of immune cells, Th_1 and Th_2 cells, which increases production of IgE and certain cytokines, predisposes people to allergies. But what causes the shift? The evidence is growing that a diet high in pro-inflammatory omega-6 fatty acids is largely to blame. Finnish researchers compared twenty allergic and twenty nonallergic mothers and found that both groups of women consumed the same amounts of omega-6 and anti-inflammatory omega-3 fatty acids in their diets. Breast milk from the allergic mothers, however, contained less of the omega-3 fatty acids, which would predispose their infants to allergies.

Long term, inhalant allergies maintain a steady inflammatory state in the body, generating free radicals that further fuel inflammation. People with inhalant allergies often have food allergies as well. Allergies are a serious stress on the body, causing unnecessary wear and tear.

Standard Treatment

Avoidance of allergens is the best way not to have allergic reactions, but it is easier accomplished when the allergen is cat dander rather than pollen. Over-the-counter antihistamine products block allergy symptoms, but at a cost: drowsiness and an increased risk of developing cancer. Some prescription antihistamines (Claritin, Allegra, and Zyrtec) are safer than others, such as Benadryl (diphenhydramine). Immunotherapy—allergy shots—can also blunt symptoms, as can corticosteroid drugs.

Perhaps the best and safest over-the-counter allergy medication is cromolyn sodium, sold under the brand name NasalCrom. Cromolyn sodium is actually a synthetic flavonoid. It works by desensitizing cells in the nasal cavity that would otherwise react to an allergen, and it appears to have no systemic side effects, as a result of being similar to the natural flavonoids in vegetables and fruit. NasalCrom is a nasal spray, and it is most effective when used several times a day, starting two weeks before pollen exposure. It may also help in dealing with allergies to cats and dogs. Other advantages of NasalCrom are that it is nonsedating and its activity appears limited to nasal tissues.

Nutrients That Can Help

Some physicians have become receptive to nutritional therapies because vitamin supplements relieved or eliminated their own allergies. For example, the late Robert Cathcart III, M.D., was impressed by how vitamin C supplements relieved his hay fever, and he went on to become one of the leading experts in the clinical use of vitamin C to fight infections.

A large variety of nutritional supplements might help, but you will have to experiment to find the best combination for your particular body and allergies. Vitamin C (1 to 5 grams daily), quercetin (300 to 1,000 mg daily), and omega-3 fish oils (1 to 3 grams daily) make a good start. Several B vitamins, including niacinamide, pantothenic acid, and vitamin B_{12}, may also help relieve allergies; a B-complex supplement may be better than individual supplements. Again, do whatever you can to reduce exposure, such as using air conditioning and high-efficiency air filters.

What Else Might Help?

Many people swear by honey as a way to reduce pollen allergies. It is very likely that honey produced in your region contains small amounts of pollen that serve as a "neutralizing dose," blocking larger amounts of pollen from triggering immune reactions.

Many foods seem to exacerbate allergic reactions to pollens, and it is probably worthwhile to test such foods by avoiding them for a week or so. Wheat, other grains, and dairy products, because of their own allergenic potential, often can aggravate pollen allergies.

Considerable research indicates that a disruption of the normal bacteria inhabiting the gastrointestinal tract can increase the likelihood of allergic sensitization during infancy. Taking antibiotics to treat ear infections is a common method of destroying normal gut bacteria. Taking probiotic (good bacteria) supplements can reduce the damage when antibiotics must be used.

The eating habits of a pregnant woman certainly influence the development of allergies in her baby. One study, published in 2008 in the *Journal of Allergy and Clinical Immunology*, of pregnant women who took supplements of *Lactobacillus rhamnosus* (one species of "good" intestinal bacteria), found that when their babies were also later given the supplements for two years, the babies were half as likely to develop skin allergies. Yet another study, published in *Archives of Disease in Childhood*, found that Swedish babies who consumed fish at an early age had a one-fourth lower risk of developing skin allergies.

Alzheimer's Disease

What Is Alzheimer's Disease?

Alzheimer's disease is the most common type of dementia. (The second most common form is caused by blood clots from ministrokes, a cardiovascular problem.) Alzheimer's is characterized by a serious impairment and worsening of memory, plus a decline in at least one other cognitive function, such as in perception or language skills. As Alzheimer's progresses, it leads to a loss of motor skills and reduced independence in daily activities, such as grooming and going to the bathroom.

Causes

Alzheimer's is characterized by deposits of beta-amyloid protein, as well as beta-amyloid tangles between brain cells. The beta-amyloid protein is believed, in some way, to choke brain cells.

How Common Is Alzheimer's Disease?

An estimated 4.5 million Americans have some degree of Alzheimer's disease. The Alzheimer Foundation projects that more than 14 million people will develop it by 2050, largely a consequence of 76 million aging baby boomers. Although these numbers may be inflated, the number of Alzheimer's cases is likely to increase because of the aging population and a decline in dietary quality.

The Inflammation Syndrome Connection

A major clue is that both animal and human studies have shown that use of ibuprofen, a common anti-inflammatory drug, reduces the risk of developing Alzheimer's disease. In animals, the drug reduces the amount of beta-amyloid plaque. People who take ibuprofen are less likely to develop the disease.

Free radicals are known to stimulate the accumulation of beta-amyloid protein, and antioxidants have been suggested by Denham Harman, M.D., Ph.D., of the University of Nebraska, as one means of counteracting the process. Of course, free radicals promote the activity of adhesion molecules in inflammation. Unfortunately, it has been difficult for researchers to document the presence of specific immune cells in the brain, which would confirm the role of inflammation.

Standard Treatment

Several drugs are used to slow the progression of Alzheimer's disease, including selegiline. Vitamin E, however, appears to be slightly more effective than selegiline.

Nutrients That Can Help

The role of free radicals in promoting brain damage points to the potential benefits of antioxidant supplements. Indeed, a range of studies with cells, animals, and people has found antioxidants to be of benefit. The most dramatic study, published in the *New England Journal of Medicine*, found that very high doses of vitamin E (2,000 IU daily) extended the ability of late-stage Alzheimer's patients to care for themselves. Researchers are currently investigating whether the same dosage of vitamin E can slow or reverse the early stages of Alzheimer's. If your mind is in good shape, however, 400 to 800 IU is probably sufficient for long-term prevention.

A number of other antioxidant supplements might also be protective, including vitamin C, coenzyme Q_{10}, and alpha-lipoic acid. Specific dosages are hard to determine because of the limited amount of research on these antioxidants and Alzheimer's disease. Extracts of the herb Ginkgo biloba might also be beneficial, although the research has been conflicting. Ginkgo serves as both an antioxidant and a dilator of blood vessels in the brain, improving blood circulation to neurons.

Some research indicates that the anti-inflammatory properties of omega-3 fish oils can also reduce the risk of neuroinflammation. Given the progressive nature of Alzheimer's disease, the emphasis should be on prevention or reversing its early stages. It is not likely that advanced Alzheimer's disease can be reversed because of extensive damage to brain cells. In a clinical trial, researchers at the Karolinska Institute, Sweden, gave omega-3 fish oils (1.7 grams of DHA and 0.6 gram EPA) to 174 men and women with Alzheimer's disease. Patients suffering from mild (but not severe) cognitive impairment improved during six months of supplementation.

Recent research points to the benefits of several other nutrients in reducing the risk of cognitive decline and Alzheimer's disease. A study published in *Archives of Internal Medicine* found that men who took beta-carotene supplements for an average of eighteen years scored much higher on cognitive tests compared with men who had been taking placebos. Beta-carotene had no short-term benefits in cognitive function. In addition, phosphatidylserine helps in normal communication between brain cells, and supplements have been shown to reverse age-related memory loss.

In 2008, researchers reported that low levels of vitamin B_{12} were strongly associated with brain shrinkage, a risk factor for developing Alzheimer's disease. Low levels of vitamin B_{12} occasionally mimic dementia. Histamine-3 receptor (H_2) antagonists (e.g., Tagamet and Zantac) interfere with vitamin B_{12} absorption and could conceivably predispose some people to develop Alzheimer's disease. Finally, curcumin enhances the ability of white blood cells to scavenge for beta-amyloid plaque. People who eat a lot of curry containing turmeric (the spice from which curcumin is obtained), have a relatively low risk of developing Alzheimer's disease.

What Else Might Help?

Several other nutrients might also protect against cognitive decline and Alzheimer's disease. Acetyl-L-carnitine, 2 grams daily, has been found to improve attention span, long-term memory, and verbal abilities in some Alzheimer's patients. Phosphatidylserine, a phosphorus-containing fat, is essential for the health of cell membranes, particularly brain cells. Dosages of 300 mg daily have been found helpful in improving memory, but 100 mg also might work in mild cases of memory impairment.

Difficulty in concentrating—that is, fuzzy thinking—is often an early sign of diabetes. Elevated blood sugar levels and full-blown diabetes accelerate the aging process and, presumably, that of the brain as well. The AI Diet Plan is a low-glycemic, glucose-stabilizing diet, and it should improve glucose tolerance.

Last but not least, it is of paramount importance to avoid abusing alcohol. Although some evidence has found that a glass or two of red wine daily lowers the risk of developing cardiovascular disease, the benefits disappear with the consumption of larger amounts of wine and especially with any regular consumption of spirit alcohols (such as whiskey, vodka, rum, and so on). First, large amounts of alcohol are toxic to the brain. Second, alcohol abusers generally are not mindful of their eating habits, producing another negative influence on the brain chemistry. Alcohol abuse can lead to the premature onset of Alzheimer's disease.

Arthritis, Osteoarthritis

What Is Osteoarthritis?

Of more than one hundred types of arthritis, osteoarthritis is by far the most common. Osteoarthritis refers specifically to a breakdown of the cartilage pad in at least one joint, such as the fingers, the knees, or the elbows. It can also affect the neck, the hips, and the lower back, even resulting in a decrease in height. These pads, known as articular cartilage, cushion the impact and lubricate the movement of bones in a joint. When articular cartilage is thin or completely gone, bones grind directly against one another. Signs of osteoarthritis include inflammation, swelling, pain, stiffness, and difficulty moving one or more joints. Nearly every person over age sixty has some degree of osteoarthritis, although the disease progresses at a different rate from person to person.

Causes

For the most part, osteoarthritis is a disease of wear and tear; the more you use your joints, the more you lose them. Overuse, such as in athletics, and athletic injuries can accelerate the breakdown of articular cartilage. Sometimes immune cells inflaming tendons can spread out and affect a nearby joint.

Being overweight, even by as few as ten pounds, can also increase the risk of osteoarthritis. One reason is that the extra weight puts more stress on joints. Another is that fat cells secrete large amounts of pro-inflammatory interleukin-6 and C-reactive protein, which increase inflammation throughout the body.

An often overlooked cause is that relatively few people nowadays consume cartilage, which contains the building blocks of our own joints. In the past, it was common to make soups using chicken or beef bones, with cartilage (and other nutrients, such as calcium) dissolving in the broth. Cartilage attached to the bones releases glucosamine and chondroitin, two important building blocks of our own cartilage. It is very possible that people would have less need for glucosamine and chondroitin supplements if they regularly consumed homemade soups.

The omega-3 fatty acids found in fish oils inhibit some of the enzymes involved in breaking down articular cartilage, so eating less fish may also increase the risk of developing osteoarthritis. In addition, aller-gylike food sensitivities may influence symptoms of osteoarthritis. Exposure to allergens often varies, and this could explain why many arthritics feel better or worse from day to day.

How Common Is Osteoarthritis?

About three times as many women as men have osteoarthritis, and about one in every fourteen people (21 million in the United States) suffer mild to crippling symptoms. That number is expected to rise to 30 million by 2020. Overall, one in seven people has some form of arthritis, 40 million in the United States. That number is expected to increase to one in six by 2020.

The Inflammation Syndrome Connection

Immune cells are drawn to sites of injury, where they release powerful inflammatory compounds. Immune cells help clean up damaged cells, such as in torn ligaments, strained tendons, and flakes of bone and cartilage. Many mild injuries may not even be noticed, or their complete healing may be wrongly assumed. Injured tissue is more susceptible to repeated injury, and this situation may lead to chronic inflammation.

Standard Treatment

More than 250 different drugs are used to treat arthritis, including aspirin and other nonsteroidal anti-inflammatory drugs (NSAIDs), cortico-steroids, and Cox-2 inhibitors. All have undesirable side effects. Some NSAIDs, such as ibuprofen, actually increase the breakdown of cartilage. Replacements of hip and knee joints are surgical treatments for severe cases of osteoarthritis.

Nutrients That Can Help

For osteoarthritis, supplements of glucosamine and chondroitin, about 1,200 to 1,500 mg of each daily, have been shown to reduce pain and inflammation. One excellent study found that glucosamine supplements can help rebuild articular cartilage, and chondroitin appears to have some anti-inflammatory properties. (For more details, review chapter 11.) Vitamin C is needed for the formation of collagen and cartilage, as are manganese and sulfur. A minimum of 500 mg of vitamin C may be needed. Additional sulfur, also essential for cartilage formation, can be obtained in glucosamine sulfate, chondroitin sulfate, or methylsulfonyl-methane (MSM), and small amounts of manganese can be obtained in a multimineral supplement.

What Else Might Help?

A variety of other nutrients, herbs, and healthy habits may also reduce the inflammation and the pain associated with osteoarthritis. The least expensive change is to drink more water. According to Hugh D. Riordan, M.D., of the Center for the Improvement of Human Functioning International, Wichita, Kansas, poor hydration is a common problem. Sufficient water intake helps cushion cells and tissues.

Vitamin D may indirectly reduce the risk of developing osteoporosis, according to research by Timothy E. McAlindon, D.M., a medical doctor and rheumatologist at Boston University Medical Center. Vitamin D is necessary for normal bone development, and low levels may affect bone structure and stability underneath the cartilage pads in joints.

Another study, by Margaret A. Flynn, Ph.D., a professor emeritus at the University of Missouri, Columbia, found that supplemental vitamin

B_{12} and folic acid could improve hand-grip strength in men and women who had osteoarthritis of the hands.

The herb ginger may also be helpful. A study in *Arthritis & Rheumatism* found that patients taking a ginger extract showed moderate improvements in knee pain. The study confirmed ginger's use as an anti-inflammatory agent in Chinese medicine, dating back more than 2,500 years.

Two topical treatments can also help. Several studies have found that creams containing capsaicin, the pungent component of hot peppers, can reduce the pain of osteoarthritis. Capsaicin blocks the transmission of pain chemicals to the brain. The effect appears to be strictly symptomatic, but other than a local sensation of heat, it is far safer than acetaminophen and other nonsteroidal anti-inflammatory drugs. Creams containing the herb arnica may also relieve joint pain.

Finally, mild movement therapies such as walking, yoga, and swimming may improve flexibility and reduce pain. It is very important, however, not to overdo such exercises because they may further break down articular cartilage.

Arthritis, Rheumatoid

What Is Rheumatoid Arthritis?

Rheumatoid arthritis is an autoimmune disease, which means that the immune system mounts a full-scale attack on the body's own tissues. In rheumatoid arthritis, the attack is centered on connective tissue near joints. Early symptoms include inflammation, pain, stiffness, tenderness, and swelling. This disease also has wide-ranging systemic effects, however, such as fever, reduced appetite, weight loss, and fatigue.

Rheumatoid arthritis is generally progressive—it gets worse with time. There may be periods of remission when symptoms decrease or even temporarily disappear. Long term, it can be disfiguring and can turn fingers into stiff, twisted digits. About 20 percent of people with rheumatoid arthritis develop lumpy nodules under the skin. In some cases, the disease becomes completely disabling.

Causes

It is possible that some cases of rheumatoid arthritis are triggered by an immune response to a viral infection. Whatever the triggering event, the severity of the disease reflects a highly disturbed immune system that cannot distinguish friendly cells from foes. To many observers, it looks as though immune cells are chasing after biochemical ghosts.

People with rheumatoid arthritis are commonly deficient in multiple nutrients. These deficiencies can impair immune function, and the benefits of nutritional supplementation have been confirmed by numerous studies. Several cases of scurvy (extreme vitamin C deficiency) have been reported with rheumatism as the most obvious symptom. Low levels of vitamin C lead to a weakening of blood vessel walls, allowing red blood cells to leak into surrounding tissue, where they trigger an immune response. Vitamin C supplementation resolved the symptoms in these patients.

How Common Is Rheumatoid Arthritis?

An estimated 2.5 million Americans (about 1 percent of the U.S. population) have rheumatoid arthritis. It affects twice as many women as men.

The Inflammation Syndrome Connection

Levels of several pro-inflammatory cytokines—interleukin-1, interleukin-6, and tumor necrosis factor alpha—are typically elevated in people with rheumatoid arthritis. These cytokines instruct immune cells to unleash a powerful attack. The tenderness, pain, and swelling are byproducts of chronic, intense inflammation.

Standard Treatment

Most medications—more than 250 different kinds—are designed to relieve pain. None of them treat the underlying disease process.

Nutrients That Can Help

Many people benefit from the anti-inflammatory effect of omega-3 fish oils; however, it may take several months to see an improvement. A Scottish study of sixty-four men and women found that taking supplements that contained about 3 grams of omega-3 fish oils daily resulted in a significant reduction of arthritic symptoms and less need to take conventional medications. Other research has shown that omega-3 fish oils reduce levels of the pro-inflammatory cytokines interleukin-1 and tumor necrosis factor alpha.

Gamma-linolenic acid (GLA), an omega-6 fatty acid that acts more like an anti-inflammatory omega-3, may be even more effective in treating rheumatoid arthritis. GLA boosts levels of anti-inflammatory pro-staglandin E_1, which suppresses pro-inflammatory prostaglandin E_2. Human trials with GLA (approximately 1.4 grams daily) have shown consistent benefits over several months, reducing symptoms by roughly one-third to one-half. Of course, results will vary from person to person, and a combination of supplements will likely have greater benefits.

Increased intake of olive oil can also ameliorate symptoms of rheumatoid arthritis. Olive oil reduces the activity of adhesion mole-cules, which enable white blood cells to attach to and attack normal cells.

People with rheumatoid arthritis tend to have low antioxidant levels, and two studies so far have found that natural vitamin E supplements sig-nificantly alleviate symptoms of the disease. The dosage used in these studies was relatively high, 1,800 IU daily. Vitamin E also lowers levels of interleukin-6 and C-reactive protein, both of which promote inflam-mation. Selenium, another antioxidant, also might help, but the research has not been consistent. The mineral boosts production of glutathione peroxidase, one of the body's main antioxidants.

People with arthritis have low levels of numerous other nutrients, such as vitamins B_2, B_6, and B_{12}; folic acid; calcium; and zinc. Deficien-cies of folic acid and vitamin B_{12} are often exacerbated by methotrexate, one of the drugs used to treat rheumatoid arthritis. Methotrexate inter-feres with the metabolism of these two B vitamins.

In 2008, doctors studied thirty-six women with rheumatoid arthritis and low blood levels of potassium. They were treated with conventional medications, along with either 6,000 mg of potassium chloride dissolved in grape juice or placebo drinks for twenty-eight days. Forty-four percent of the women receiving supplemental potassium had a significant decrease in arthritic pain, and 31 percent had a moderate reduction in pain, according to an article in the *Journal of Pain*. The dose of potas-sium was large, and you should not take it without a prescription and clear direction from your physician (to minimize the risk of heart-rhythm abnormalities). A safe alternative to potassium supplements is to con-sume potassium-rich foods, including coconut water (not coconut milk). One unsweetened 11-ounce container of coconut water provides 660 mg of potassium.

What Else Might Help?

Many studies point to the apparent role of allergylike food sensitivities in rheumatoid arthritis. These adverse reactions to food can ramp up immune activity and inflammation. Dairy products and gluten-containing grains (such as wheat, rye, and barley) are among the most common food allergens, and studies have found that avoiding them eases arthritic symptoms, such as morning stiffness and the number of swollen joints in many people, as well as reducing C-reactive protein levels. The elimination of allergenic foods may explain why fasting and gluten-free vegetarian diets help some people with rheumatoid arthritis.

According to Loren Cordain, Ph.D., a researcher at Colorado State University, lectins might also trigger symptoms of rheumatoid arthritis in some people. Lectins are a family of plant proteins found primarily in legumes but also in wheat and rice. Like gluten, lectins may cause an inflammation of the gut, leading to a more generalized immune response. Temporarily avoiding lectin-containing foods may help you confirm a sensitivity to them.

Two additional supplements might also be of benefit: An animal study found that the antioxidant extract of green tea blocked the activity of several pro-inflammatory compounds, protecting against rheumatoid arthritis. Other research suggests that supplemental cetyl-myristoleate might lessen symptoms of rheumatoid arthritis as well.

Asthma

What Is Asthma?

During asthmatic episodes, or attacks, the body's airways (bronchi and bronchioles, which deliver air to the lungs) overreact to pollen, cat dander, cigarette smoke, cold air, or other stimuli. The airway wall muscles begin to spasm, narrowing the opening and allowing less air to reach the lungs. An inflammatory response results in a rapid thickening of mucus, which further narrows the airway. An asthma attack may begin with wheezing, coughing, or shortness of breath; suffocation can occur in rare cases.

Causes

Ask ten different allergists about the cause of asthma and you may get twenty different explanations. A nearly mind-boggling number of causes have been proposed: dust, dust mites, cockroaches, house mice, wall-to-wall carpeting, central heating, gas stoves, overly sealed (insulated) buildings, *Candida* yeast infections, pollen, and food allergies. In addition, some people blame urban air pollution. Although air pollution certainly can trigger asthmatic attacks, urban air pollution has generally declined, while the number of people with asthma has increased. The same pattern is true with secondhand cigarette smoke, which can increase the risk of asthma in children—but fewer people are smoking, and the rate of asthma continues to rise. Others point the finger at the widespread use of antibacterial cleansers or antibiotics, both of which might reduce routine exposures to bacteria and interfere with the normal programming of immune systems.

All of the previous factors can trigger asthmatic reactions in sensitive people. So can a host of other factors, such as exercise, cold air, aspirin, sulfites (a preservative used in wines, beers, and some salad bars), and tartrazine (a yellow coloring used in some foods and drugs). In addition, emotional stress can induce asthmatic reactions in some people, and being overweight predisposes some people to asthma.

Like a fish that does not realize it is living in polluted waters, many people with asthma and many allergists don't understand that they are essentially swimming in a polluted diet. The modern diet, which is high in pro-inflammatory omega-6 and trans-fatty acids and low in antioxidants, sets the stage for asthmatic reactions. In effect, asthma is one of many diseases of modern civilization and modern eating habits.

People with asthma tend to have higher than normal levels of free radicals, which stimulate inflammatory reactions and also indicate a low intake of antioxidant nutrients. Several studies have found that both children and adults have better lung function and are less likely to wheeze when they eat a lot of fruits and vegetables, the main dietary sources of antioxidants. Breast-feeding may also reduce the risk of developing asthma and other respiratory illnesses. J. Stewart Forsyth, M.D., of Ninewells Hospital, Dundee, Scotland, noted in the *British Medical Journal* that "nutritional deficiencies at critical periods of fetal and infant growth may induce permanent changes in physiological function."

Other research points to inadequate levels of anti-inflammatory omega-3 fish oils in the diet. A study of almost six hundred children by Ann J. Woolcock, M.D., of the Royal Prince Alfred Hospital, Australia, found that those who regularly ate fresh fish that were rich in omega-3 fatty acids had one-fourth the risk of getting asthma, compared with children who ate little or no fish. In a separate article, Jennifer K. Peat, Ph.D., a colleague of Woolcock's, noted that the increase of childhood asthma corresponded with a fivefold increase in the use of vegetable oils (rich in pro-inflammatory omega-6 fatty acids) and a shift to using margarine instead of butter. Similar changes have occured in New Zealand, England, and the United States.

How Common Is Asthma?

Asthma is the most common *obstructive airway disease*. Several decades ago, it was a rare respiratory disorder. Today it affects 22 million Americans, one-third of them children. Its prevalence in the United States has doubled since the 1970s, and African Americans and Hispanics experience particularly high rates of the disease. In Britain, the incidence of asthma in children doubled during the 1990s.

The Inflammation Syndrome Connection

Asthma usually begins when the immune system becomes sensitized to an allergen, which may be a food, tobacco, proteins from cockroach feces, or dander from pets. The immune system responds whether the trigger is a real threat or not, releasing a variety of inflammatory molecules. An upper respiratory tract reaction may cause little more than a runny nose (rhinitis), but asthma develops when the bronchi or bronchioles (which branch out from the bronchi) start overreacting to inflammatory molecules. One relationship is clear: the increase in asthma is related to the overall surge in allergies—that is, inflammatory reactions to generally innocuous substances.

Standard Treatment

A wide variety of medications are used to lessen asthmatic reactions, including corticosteroids and bronchial dilators. Most have long-term consequences. For example, corticosteroids increase the risk of developing cataracts and weak bones.

Nutrients That Can Help

Several studies have shown that consuming large amounts of antioxidant nutrients can greatly reduce the frequency and severity of asthmatic reactions. Herman A. Cohen, M.D., of Rabin Medical Center, Israel, gave 2 grams of vitamin C or a placebo to twenty men and women, ages seven to twenty-eight, all with exercise-induced asthma. An hour after they took the vitamin or the placebo, their lung function was measured as they walked or ran on a treadmill. Half of the patients had milder asthmatic reactions after taking the vitamin C, while those taking placebos experienced a significant decline in lung function.

Similarly, researchers at the University of Washington, Seattle, gave vitamin E (400 IU) and vitamin C (500 mg) daily to patients with asthma who were exposed to ozone (an air pollutant) and were asked to run on a treadmill. After taking the antioxidants, the patients tolerated the ozone and the exercise with considerably less breathing difficulty and, sometimes, with improvements in lung function.

Two studies have found that the antioxidants beta-carotene and lycopene, found in vegetables and fruit, can ease asthmatic reactions. Ami Ben-Amotz, Ph.D., of Israel's National Institute of Oceanography, and his colleagues measured lung function in thirty-eight people with asthma, then asked them to run on a treadmill. The subjects had an average decrease of at least 15 percent in their lung function. Next, Ben-Amotz gave them 64 mg of natural beta-carotene (derived from *Dunaliella* algae) daily for seven days. After taking the supplements (equivalent to about 100,000 IU daily), they went back on the treadmill. This time, twenty (53 percent) of the subjects had significant improvements in their postexercise breathing. In particular, these twenty patients initially had an average 25 percent decrease in lung function after exercising, but only a 5 percent reduction after taking beta-carotene supplements.

In the other study, Ben-Amotz asked twenty people with exercise-induced asthma to take either 30 mg of lycopene (the amount found in seven tomatoes) or placebos daily for one week. All of the subjects taking placebos had a 15 percent decline in lung function after exercising. But 55 percent of those taking lycopene had improvements in lung function after exercising.

Ozone, a common component of urban air pollution, is toxic to the respiratory system, and it increases the inflammatory response in people with asthma. In a study at the University of Washington, Seattle, however, taking supplements of vitamin E (400 IU) and vitamin C (500 mg) daily greatly improved breathing in seventeen adults with asthma after they were exposed to ozone.

In addition, research has found that omega-3 fatty acids—3 grams daily—can significantly reduce bronchial reactivity in asthmatic patients. Other studies have found similar benefits, although the results have not always been uniform. Rather than relying only on omega-3 fatty acids, people with asthma might have greater success by also taking gamma-linolenic acid, vitamin E, and other nutritional supplements.

The most recent nutrition research points to benefits from two supplements, Pycnogenol and gamma-linolenic acid. In a study of children with asthma, taking Pycnogenol supplements improved lung function, and many of the children were able to decrease or stop using their medications. Meanwhile, a study of adults found that a combination of gamma-linolenic acid and fish oils led to a reduction in asthma symptoms. Gamma-linolenic acid specifically cuts down on the production of leukotrienes, a family of pro-inflammatory molecules involved in asthma.

What Else Might Help?

Many other nutrients help ease asthmatic reactions, and it is worth trying them—in addition to strictly following the AI Diet Plan. People with asthma commonly have low levels of magnesium, a mineral involved in more than three hundred biochemical processes in the body. Magnesium is also a mild muscle relaxant, so it may directly reduce the frequency and severity of reactions. In addition, zinc and selenium might be of benefit, along with quercetin (which inhibits some types of inflammation-promoting adhesion molecules) and the herb boswellia. A study published in the *Journal of Medicinal Food* reported that the herbal antioxidant Pycnogenol (1 mg per pound of body weight, up to 200 mg daily) improved lung function in patients with asthma. It is also important to maintain a normal weight, because being overweight increases the risk of asthma. (See the section "Overweight and Obesity" in this chapter.)

Athletic and Other Injuries

What Are Athletic Injuries?

Athletic injuries can damage tissues so severely that they ultimately lead to chronic inflammation and pain and a complete breakdown of those tissues. The same can happen for any type of nonathletic physical injury as well, such as a broken bone from a fall or a muscle strain from lifting too heavy an object. Experiencing pain and discomfort long after an injury are signs of its incomplete healing.

Most athletic injuries and other types of physical injuries affect the skin, the cartilage, the muscles, and the bones. Muscle strains and sprains, tendinitis, and bone fractures are the most common injuries. Repeated stress to the cartilage pads in joints, particularly in the knees, can weaken these cushions and set the stage for osteoarthritis. Physical stresses may also bruise internal organs such as the kidneys or the brain. For example, many boxers develop neurological damage years after they fought in the ring and absorbed punches. Even marathon runners exhibit elevated levels of inflammation-causing substances after a long-distance run.

Causes

Serious single injuries, repeated bruising, and overuse injuries are physical stresses to the body. They crush, tear, or break tissues, and healed tissue may not be quite as sturdy or resilient as tissue that has never been injured. Granted, accidental injuries are sometimes unavoidable, regardless of whether a person is a well-conditioned athlete or an average person who happens to trip over a crack in the sidewalk.

Injuries generate large numbers of free radicals that are released by activated white blood cells. Studies have found that broken bones and damaged cartilage increase free-radical levels, even without the presence of white blood cells. In addition, ischemic-reperfusion injuries boost free-radical levels and tissue damage. Ischemia refers to a reduction of blood flow, often the first phase of an injury, which is followed by an influx of red blood cells; both phases generate large quantities of free radicals.

In general, the risk of suffering injuries and undergoing painfully slow healing increases with age. Everyone knows that children tend to bounce back from injuries, but adults heal much more slowly. As was discussed earlier, our bodies experience an age-related deterioration. Bones, skin, and other tissues become thinner, and muscle mass declines—these are, after all, some of the signs of aging. It is important to keep in mind that fifty-year-olds don't have the physical attributes of twenty-five-year-olds. The chances of being injured can increase when a person denies the reality of aging and its concomitant decreases in strength, flexibility, reflexes, and coordination. When injuries occur, it is imperative that chronic inflammation be prevented and healing be supported nutritionally.

How Common Are Athletic Injuries?

Every person involved in athletic activities risks some type of injury. Professional athletes are conditioned and trained to minimize the chances of suffering such injuries, but injuries still occur. For example, professional baseball pitchers usually rest for at least three days after a game. Weekend warriors, people who engage in sports only occasionally, are often neither conditioned nor trained. They run a high risk of developing overuse injuries, such as tennis elbow, golf elbow, or sore knees, as well as far more serious injuries.

The Inflammation Syndrome Connection

Inflammation is the body's immediate response to injury. It enables a variety of blood cells to flood the site of the injury—platelets to stop bleeding, red blood cells to nourish healthy cells, and white blood cells to clear up damaged cells and fight infections. Without adequate levels of many nutrients, however, healing cannot be completed and the inflammatory response cannot be turned off.

Standard Treatment

NSAIDs are commonly used to reduce inflammation and pain, but they can lead to excessive bleeding and ulcers. Some injuries must be treated surgically.

Nutrients That Can Help

The omega-3 fish oils, particularly eicosapentaenoic acid (EPA), are very helpful in resolving athletic injuries. In particular, high-EPA fish oil supplements can reduce delayed-onset muscle soreness (DOMS), which typically develops several hours after intense exercise. Contrary to what many athletes believe, DOMS is not caused by lactic acid production. Rather, it results from microscopic tears to muscle fibers, followed by inflammation, swelling, and pain. EPA reduces prostaglandin E_2, a principal cause of both inflammation and pain. One of the high-EPA products I recommend specifically for athletes is Recoup 90 (www.recoup90.com). The German Olympic Weight Lifting Team used this product as a food supplement during the 2008 Olympics in Beijing.

Many athletes also experience overuse injuries that cause inflammation and pain for several weeks. Conventional treatments usually require that athletes refrain from workouts during this extended recovery period, but this is difficult for elite athletes who are used to consistent physical activity and want to stay in top form. To speed healing from overuse injuries and to allow elite athletes to continue training during recovery, the Danish Olympic team frequently relies on PharmaNord's Bio-Sport, which combines large amounts of omega-3 fish oils and gamma-linolenic acid. The product is available in Europe but not in the United States. I do recommend a similar product, Carlson's Inflammation Balance (www.carlsonlabs.com), which is available in the United States.

Søren Mavrogenis, a physiotherapist in Copenhagen and the chief physical therapist for the Danish Olympic team, regularly uses Bio-Sport to treat overuse injuries in Olympians and other athletes. The product provides 706 mg of omega-3 fish oils, 670 mg of gamma-linolenic acid, and modest amounts of antioxidant vitamins and minerals daily. If you cannot purchase Bio-Sport, simply buy other products and round off the dosages. You will achieve comparable benefits.

In one of several controlled studies, Søren and Norwegian physicians treated forty recreational athletes, men and women eighteen to sixty years old, with the fatty acid/antioxidant supplement or placebos for one month. All of the subjects had suffered overuse injuries in sports activities and experienced chronic inflammation for at least three months before entering the study. In addition to the supplements and the placebos, the subjects also received physical therapy. Nearly all of the participants had significant reductions in their inflammation and pain.

Exercise is well documented for increasing levels of free radicals, which can damage DNA. This DNA damage may account for the weathered looks of many serious athletes. Clinical trials have found that vitamin E supplements can reduce or prevent such DNA damage. Vitamin C quenches free radicals as well and is also crucial for forming new collagen and cartilage during the healing process.

What Else Might Help?

Pycnogenol, a complex of natural antioxidants obtained from the bark of French maritime pine trees, has impressive anti-inflammatory properties. It also increases the body's synthesis of collagen and elastin, another tissue protein. Anthony Martin, D.C., of Montreal, has advised many professional Canadian athletes who have been injured. In one case, a hockey player who had injured his knee was told by his team's physician that he would probably need surgery and would be on the sidelines for eight weeks. Martin recommended that the player take 400 mg daily of Pycnogenol. His knee stopped swelling, and after a week he no longer needed crutches. He was also able to avoid surgery and was playing hockey again after only three weeks.

Several other nutrients may be especially helpful in healing injuries. Methylsulfonylmethane (MSM), 1,000 to 2,000 mg daily, has been found very effective in reducing muscle and joint pain. S-adenosyl-L-methionine (SAMe) stimulates the body's production of collagen. Both nutrients likely work at least in part because they donate sulfur to key biochemical processes. In addition, the B vitamins have an analgesic effect and are required for the production of new, healthy cells.

I also recommend arnica, an herb long used to reduce muscle soreness and bruising. It seems to work best when applied immediately after injuries. My favorite arnica product is Arnicare, made by Boiron. It comes in a tube and is intended to be a topical rub.

Cancer

What Is Cancer?

Cancer refers to the growth of abnormal cells, which can displace the normal cells that compose tissues. Cancers are often distinguished by their ability to metastasize, spreading to and attacking other organs. There are many different types of cancer, but all arouse fear because of how they cut life expectancy and because of the pain associated with cancer and with conventional therapies (surgery, radiation, and chemotherapy). Although some cancers affect children, they are usually age-related: the older you are, the greater your risk of getting cancer. In general, cancers take years to develop, and many cancers go undiagnosed until an autopsy is performed on the deceased person.

Causes

Cancers are caused by mutations, or changes, in the deoxyribonucleic acid (DNA) that programs cell behavior. These mutations generally occur in two ways: through random transcriptional errors when cells normally replicate, and through free-radical damage to DNA. These errors permanently alter the cells' genetic instructions, which is analogous to being told to turn right on a street instead of left. The immune system recognizes and destroys most abnormal cells, but some are able to evade normal immunity. As a person gets older, a larger number of cell mutations and poor immune surveillance increase the likelihood of cancer.

How Common Is Cancer?

Cancer is now the leading cause of death in the United States and one of the most common causes of death worldwide. A little more than five hundred thousand Americans die of cancer each year. By far, cancers of the lungs and the bronchi are the leading causes of cancer-related deaths in the United States, and they are also a common cause of death among nonsmokers. Breast cancer in women, prostate cancer in men, and colorectal cancer are the next most common types of cancer. In children, brain cancer has replaced leukemia as the most common cancer.

The Inflammation Syndrome Connection

According to Bruce N. Ames, Ph.D., a leading cell biologist at the University of California, Berkeley, about 30 percent of all cancers are related to chronic inflammation or chronic infections. Both inflammation and infections generate free radicals, which can damage DNA, and the level of damage increases when these conditions are chronic. In addition, viruses can cause cells to mutate.

Standard Treatment

Conventional medical treatments of cancer are generally aggressive and are designed to eradicate cancerous cells. They include surgical removal of the tumor mass or the affected organ, radiation, and chemotherapy. Despite the many claims of advances in cancer treatment, the cure often seems worse than the disease. Indeed, an analysis published in the *Journal of the American Medical Association* found that improvements in the so-called five-year survival rate in cancer patients had more to do with better (earlier) diagnosis than with successful cures.

Nutrients That Can Help

Good nutrition and a high intake of most micronutrients help preserve the integrity of DNA. Because of this, nearly every nutrient can play an important role in reducing the risk of cancer; however, some nutrients may be more important than others.

Antioxidant nutrients curb the activity of free radicals and, as a consequence, can reduce DNA damage. Selenium, part of the potent antioxidant glutathione peroxidase, has been shown to inhibit dangerous mutations to the flu and coxsackie viruses; in addition, vitamin E prevents mutations to the coxsackie virus. Based on this research, it is highly plausible that selenium and vitamin E might block virus-induced mutations that could give rise to cancer cells.

Antioxidants, such as vitamins E and C, reduce DNA damage from various types of free radicals; however, antioxidants also play roles in cell-to-cell communication and can help direct cancer cells to self-destruct, a process that researchers call apoptosis. Considerable research now shows that high-dose vitamin C—particularly regular intravenous

50-gram infusions—lessens the risk of cancer recurrence. Some of the research, in cell and animal experiments as well as with people, has been conducted at the National Institutes for Health and other institutions and clinics around the world. These large amounts of vitamin C likely support the healing process after surgery and other treatments, which is important because many cancer patients do not heal adequately after conventional therapies.

The B vitamins play crucial roles in the body's synthesis and repair of damaged DNA. Folic acid, vitamin B_{12}, vitamin B_3, and vitamin B_1 may be particularly important, especially in ensuring accurate gene transcription and repair. Some research also suggests that the omega-3 fatty acids reduce inflammation in the digestive tract and may lessen the risk of developing colon cancer.

Over the last few years, studies of people have shown that several other nutrients, particularly in the form of supplements, can reduce the risk of developing cancer. Some supplements have striking benefits in quality of life for patients undergoing treatment and even in late-stage cancer patients. For example, some evidence (in animal studies) points to N-acetylcysteine reducing "chemo brain," the mental fogginess that often develops as a consequence of chemotherapy. Meanwhile, Korean researchers reported in 2007 that a combination of oral and intravenous vitamin C reduced pain and nausea in patients considered terminal.

European researchers recently reported that women with BRCA1 genetic mutations (which significantly increase the risk of developing breast and ovarian cancer) had abnormally high rates of mutations in immune cells. The BRCA1 gene normally enhances the repair of damaged genes, but BRCA1 mutations allow gene damage to accumulate. Within three months of the study participants' beginning supplementation with selenium, a mineral needed for antioxidant protection, the rate of mutations in these women decreased to normal levels. Meanwhile, doctors at the Karmano Cancer Institute in Detroit, Michigan, found that taking relatively large amounts (30 mg daily) of tomato-based lycopene led to a regression in prostate cancers in men scheduled for surgery.

Vitamin D, which has entered a nutrition renaissance, may provide the broadest protection against cancer. More than sixty studies have so far noted that high levels of vitamin D are associated with a reduced risk of developing several cancers, including those of the breast, the colon, and the prostate. One recent clinical trial, published in the *American Journal of Clinical Nutrition*, found that a combination of vitamin D and calcium supplements led to a 60 percent lower incidence of leukemias, myelomas, and breast, colon, lung, and lymph cancers. Unfortunately, an estimated 50 percent of Americans are deficient in vitamin D. Michael Holick, M.D., of the Boston University Medical School, and many other experts now recommend that every infant, child, and adult take at least 1,000 IU of vitamin D supplements daily.

What Else Might Help?

Cigarette smoke and other pollutants do their damage in large part by disrupting normal DNA transcription and by causing free-radical damage to DNA. Some of the free radicals may be part of the chemical pollutants; other free radicals may be produced when the liver tries to break down the pollutants. Thus, it helps to avoid tobacco smoke, to live in a city that does not have serious air pollution, and to minimize exposure to cancer-causing chemicals at work and at home. If avoidance is not possible, the evidence suggests that supplemental vitamin E, selenium, and B vitamins—along with a diet that contains a diverse selection of vegetables—might rank toward the top of a cancer-prevention strategy.

Several aspects of diet are especially relevant in this context. First, high-fat diets promote the growth of many cancers, such as those of the breast and the prostate. For prevention and during cancer treatment, it is worthwhile to reduce and, especially, to alter the ratios of specific types of fats. Several compelling studies have shown that fish oils have a cancer-suppressive effect. In contrast, corn, safflower, and other vegetable oils that are high in omega-6 fatty acids promote the growth of cancers.

In addition, researchers at the University of Utah, Salt Lake City, had determined that diets high in trans fats are associated with significant increases in the risk of colon cancer. Given the fundamental roles of fatty acids in health, it would be prudent to avoid a synthetic fat that interferes with other fatty acids. Thus, the ideal approach during cancer treatment might be to drastically reduce overall fat intake, while emphasizing fish and taking fish oil supplements. Under these circumstances, it might also be best to avoid red meats and even to limit consumption of chicken and turkey.

Two other points warrant discussion. One, high estrogen levels increase the risk of developing breast cancer, and women have a fivefold variation in their production of estrogen. Painful menstrual periods and endometriosis are signs of high estrogen, and oral contraceptives and hormone-replacement therapy may further stimulate the growth of breast and ovarian cancers. Alcohol heightens the activity of estrogen receptors on cells, increasing the potency of estrogens, and many plastics and pesticides function as estrogen mimics in the body. The B-complex vitamins, particularly choline and inositol, may help break down all of these estrogens.

Second, grapefruit and other citrus fruits contain many antioxidant flavonoids that may reduce the risk of getting cancer. Some recent research, however, suggests that grapefruit (and possibly other citrus fruits) may increase women's risk of developing breast cancer. The link is not definitive, but grapefruit does block the activity of certain liver enzymes involved in breaking down drugs and hormones. It is conceivable that women who consume large amounts of grapefruit diminish their ability to break down estrogen. As a caution, women at high risk of developing breast cancer (such as those who carry the BRCA1 or BRCA2 gene) or those who have been diagnosed with breast cancer might do well to avoid grapefruit juice.

Chronic Obstructive Pulmonary Disease

What Is Chronic Obstructive Pulmonary Disease?

Chronic obstructive pulmonary disease (COPD) is a chronic blockage of the airways, resulting from chronic bronchitis or emphysema. Chronic bronchitis is defined as a persistent cough with sputum, without a medically identifiable cause. Emphysema describes an enlargement of minute air sacs, called alveoli, and the destruction of their walls, which impair lung function. When the lungs cannot take in adequate oxygen, the body's cells become oxygen-deprived.

Causes

The leading cause of COPD is smoking, although urban air pollution can also degrade lung capacity. COPD may start to develop within five to ten years after a person starts to smoke. Smoker's cough is one sign of COPD, as is the tendency for a head cold to move to the chest. By the time a person reaches his or her late fifties or early sixties, reduced lung function may result in shortness of breath, making bathing, cooking, and dressing difficult.

How Common Is Chronic Obstructive Pulmonary Disease?

In the United States an estimated 14 million people have COPD, and approximately 104,000 die from it each year.

The Inflammation Syndrome Connection

Almost 5,000 chemicals have been identified in cigarette smoke. Many of these release free radicals, which damage the proteins (elastin and collagen) that form the matrix of lung cells. In addition, white blood cells collect in the alveoli, causing inflammation and further destruction of lung tissue. One cannot overstate the damaging effects of cigarette smoke—it is like living in a burning building and breathing in all of the noxious chemicals.

Standard Treatment

Prognosis of and treatments for COPD are limited, though moderate exercise may improve overall quality of life.

Nutrients That Can Help

Compelling evidence indicates that a number of antioxidants and omega-3 fish oils may lessen the impact of air pollutants on lungs and help maintain normal lung function. This does not prove that these nutrients might help reduce the risk or severity of COPD; however, it is likely that these nutrients would exert some benefits in COPD, as long as they were consumed long before lung damage became irreversible.

N-acetylcysteine (NAC) is sometimes used by physicians to break up mucus in the lungs. When taken on a long-term basis, NAC may help protect lung cells. A number of other antioxidants might also be helpful. Studies of smokers and beta-carotene have shown contradictory effects, but a modest intake of this carotene (10,000 IU or 6 mg) *in combination with other antioxidants*, such as vitamins E and C, is likely to be helpful. There appears to be a threshold of benefits from beta-carotene *in smokers*, so the above dosage should not be exceeded.

In a study of street workers in Mexico City, which is regarded as the most polluted large city in the world, men were asked to take 75 mg of vitamin E, 650 mg of vitamin C, and 15 mg of beta-carotene or placebos daily for 2½ months. When ozone levels were elevated, lung function in all of the men declined; however, men taking the antioxidant cocktail maintained better lung function throughout the study.

Still other research has found that lung function throughout life is related to the consumption of fruits and vegetables and the resultant high blood levels of antioxidants. One study found that vitamin E and beta-cryptoxanthin (found in papayas, peaches, tangerines, and oranges) were most strongly associated with good lung function.

James E. Gadek, M.D., of Ohio State University Medical Center, found that hospitalized patients with respiratory distress syndrome had significant improvements after they were fed a low-carbohydrate formula with vitamins E and C, beta-carotene, omega-3 fatty acids, and gamma-linolenic acid.

Some preliminary research suggests that sulforaphane, a compound found in broccoli, may restore normal antioxidant activity in lung cells. The experiments were conducted at the Johns Hopkins School of Medicine in Baltimore, Maryland. Because of the severity of COPD, a diet high in broccoli might diminish the risk of developing the disease. Smoking cessation, however, remains the ideal approach.

What Else Might Help?

There is no pill, natural or pharmaceutical, that will protect a person from the health effects of smoking. If you smoke, try your best to stop. Short of that, eat as many fruits and vegetables as you can. Smokers typically eat few fruits and vegetables, a rich and diverse source of antioxidant nutrients.

Coronary Artery (Heart) Disease

What Is Coronary Artery (Heart) Disease?

Coronary artery disease is characterized by a narrowing of the major arteries in the heart, a situation that leads to reduced blood flow and, in effect, a slow starvation of cells that form the heart. The narrowing is caused by several factors, including lesions made up of cholesterol, abnormal growth of smooth muscle cells, and accumulated platelet cells. A heart attack occurs when a lesion grows large enough to completely block blood flow to the heart or when part of a lesion breaks off and blocks an artery.

Causes

Theories describing the cause of coronary artery (heart) disease often become fashionable and then, after a number of years, unfashionable.

Elevated levels of cholesterol were long seen as a major cause of heart and other cardiovascular diseases. The cholesterol theory oversimplifies the multifactorial causes of heart disease and is being replaced by other theories, although you could not tell that by the large numbers of cholesterol-lowering drugs prescribed.

The two best explanations involve nutritional deficiencies and inflammatory injury to artery walls, and it is likely that both processes occur simultaneously. (They are not mutually exclusive.) One theory, proposed by Kilmer McCully, M.D., in 1969, argues that lack of certain B vitamins (chiefly, folic acid and vitamin B_6) disrupts a fundamental biochemical process known as methylation. As a consequence, blood levels of homocysteine increase, damaging blood vessel walls. The body's response, a misguided attempt to heal the damage, actually leads to the deposition of cholesterol, calcium, and other substances.

The other theory, which dates back in part to clinical work by Evan Shute, M.D., in the 1940s and research by Denham Harman, M.D., in the 1950s, argues that oxidized LDL cholesterol is swallowed by white blood cells, which become lodged in the matrix of cells in artery walls. More recent clinical research by a variety of researchers, including Ishwarlal "Kenny" Jialal, M.D., of the University of Texas Southwestern Medical Center, Dallas, has clearly shown that *oxidized* but not normal LDL cholesterol is attacked and engulfed by white blood cells. What makes this research so intriguing is that LDL is the medium through which fat-soluble nutrients such as vitamin E are carried in the blood. Oxidized LDL cholesterol is a sign of inadequate vitamin E intake (or, conversely, excessive intake of oxidized fats, such as in fried foods). Just as the B vitamins reduce homocysteine levels, so vitamin E reduces the oxidation of LDL cholesterol.

How Common Is Coronary Artery (Heart) Disease?

An estimated 60 million Americans have coronary artery disease, and approximately 725,000 die each year from it in the United States. It is the leading cause of death in Canada and England. Stroke accounts for another 116,000 annual deaths in the United States, with ischemic stroke (in effect, a "heart attack" in the brain) being the most common type.

The Inflammation Syndrome Connection

Research on the inflammatory nature of homocysteine and oxidized LDL cholesterol has helped establish coronary artery disease as an inflammatory process. The role of inflammation in heart disease has become better understood by the commercialization of a highly sensitive C-reactive protein (CRP) test and a shift in the medical perception of CRP. In the past, high blood levels of CRP were seen as a marker of the body's inflammatory response after traumatic injury. The view today, which is more accurate, is that CRP is also a promoter of inflammation. It is a direct by-product of interleukin-6, perhaps the most inflammatory of the cytokines.

Although CRP levels reflect a general level of inflammation in the body, elevated CRP levels are a far more reliable predictor of heart disease than either cholesterol or homocysteine is. People with high CRP levels are 4½ times more likely to experience a heart attack than are people who have normal levels. Arterial lesions containing CRP are unstable and highly likely to lead to breakaway fragments and clots. It is this relationship between CRP and heart disease, perhaps more than any other recent event, that has raised the medical consciousness of the role of inflammation in heart disease and other diseases.

Standard Treatment

The most common treatment for coronary artery disease consists of a class of cholesterol-lowering drugs known as statins. These drugs currently include Lipitor (atorvastatin), Mevacor (lovastatin), Pravachol (pravastatin), and Zocor (simvastatin). Elevated cholesterol is more a symptom than a cause of coronary artery disease, however, so these and other drugs merely alter symptoms without addressing the underlying causes. Recent studies have found that statins do reduce CRP levels; however, these drugs pose a risk of serious side effects. Surgical treatments such as bypass and balloon angioplasty are also used to correct blocked arteries but do not change the underlying disease process.

Nutrients That Can Help

Many nutrients inhibit the inflammatory process in blood vessel walls and provide a variety of improvements in heart function. Several B vitamins lower homocysteine levels and appear to reduce a person's risk of having a heart attack. One study, published in the November 29, 2001, *New England Journal of Medicine*, found that modest supplements of folic acid, vitamin B$_6$, and vitamin B$_{12}$ significantly lowered homocysteine levels and clearly reversed coronary artery disease in heart patients. Reducing homocysteine levels eliminates a major cause of blood vessel inflammation.

As discussed earlier, vitamin E supplements lower CRP levels and, several clinical trials have found, reduce the risk of heart disease and heart attack. Vitamin E also decreases the tendency of LDL cholesterol to oxidize, which in turn keeps white blood cells from attacking LDL. In addition, vitamin E prevents the stiffening of blood vessel walls (endothelial dysfunction), which lessens blood flow and increases the risk of heart disease. Vitamin E also turns off the gene that programs the growth of excess smooth muscle cells, which narrows blood vessels.

The omega-3 fatty acids found in fish oils and other sources have diverse benefits for one's health, stemming in part from their anti-inflammatory and cytokine-modulating properties. Research has found that the omega-3 fatty acids can reduce heart irregularities known as cardiac arrhythmias and can also lower blood pressure. In 2001, Danish researchers reported in the *American Journal of Cardiology* that heart patients with extensive narrowing of blood vessels had elevated levels of CRP and had low levels of omega-3 fatty acids. Supplements of omega-3 fatty acids should always be taken with vitamin E to protect them against oxidation.

Vitamin C and the B vitamin niacin (a form of B_3, which causes a temporary flushing sensation) have been found to lower cholesterol levels and to lower levels of lipoprotein (a), a cholesterol fraction that increases the risk of developing heart disease. In addition, magnesium plays a crucial role in regulating heart rhythm, and supplements can sometimes reduce arrhythmias.

Over the last few years, three other nutrients have been found helpful in reducing the risk of developing coronary artery disease. People with high blood levels of vitamin D, from either supplements or regular sun exposure, are less likely to develop heart disease or heart failure. L-arginine, a building block of protein, is needed to make nitric oxide, a chemical that regulates blood vessel tone and can lower blood pressure. Finally, one of the two forms of vitamin K_2 (the MK-7 form, 100 to 200 mcg daily) may reduce coronary calcification, also known as hardening of the arteries. Vitamin K is contraindicated, however, for people taking Coumadin (warfarin) or other blood-thinning drugs that reduce vitamin K activity.

What Else Might Help?

It is of utmost importance to follow a diet that emphasizes nutrient density, such as the AI Diet Plan, which stresses fish, lean meats, and large amounts of fresh vegetables. Diets high in refined carbohydrates, sugars, and partially hydrogenated vegetable oils set the stage for insulin resistance and overweight, which increase the risk of developing pre- and full-blown diabetes and heart disease. Such a dietary approach, combined with anti-inflammatory nutritional supplements, also should reduce the severity of phlebitis, varicose veins, and blood pressure.

Finding some means of stress reduction or stress management is important as well. Stress raises levels of cortisol, which in turn boosts insulin levels—contributing to an increased risk of both abdominal obesity and heart disease. Removing yourself from the stress, even temporarily, can have an extraordinary effect. Consider a daily walk (which also lowers glucose and insulin levels), meditation, a hobby, recreational reading, or sightseeing as a stress-reducing activity.

Dental Inflammation

What Is Dental Inflammation?

Three common dental disorders involve significant levels of inflammation: gingivitis, periodontitis, and temporomandibular joint (TMJ) syndrome. Chronic gingivitis refers to inflammation in the gum tissues that are visible near the teeth. If your gums bleed when you floss or brush your teeth, there is a good chance that you have gingivitis. Periodontitis describes inflammation that is much deeper and involves the supporting bone of the teeth, and it is often missed in casual examinations. Periodontitis erodes the bone that forms teeth. TMJ syndrome is generally recognized as a misalignment of the temporomandibular joint, located near the ears, which hinges the jawbone to the skull. This misalignment generates free radicals, which can fuel inflammation.

Causes

Each of these disorders has a different cause. Gingivitis results in large part from poor dental hygiene, which allows plaque-causing bacteria to proliferate and attack the gums. Periodontitis is associated with a different type of bacteria, but it is also often an age-related condition because some bone loss increases with age. TMJ syndrome is generally considered a consequence of malocclusion (crooked teeth); however, the educator and author Malcolm Riley, D.D.S., of London, England, believes that TMJ syndrome is caused largely by stress, which leads to TMJ muscular spasms and pain.

How Common Is Dental Inflammation?

Dental caries (cavities) and periodontitis affect nearly every person at some point in life. For example, three out of four people develop some degree of gum disease by age thirty-five. The American Dental Association estimates that 10 million people in the United States might suffer from some amount of TMJ disease.

The Inflammation Syndrome Connection

In gingivitis, inflammation develops in response to bacterial infiltration of the gums. Similarly, in periodontitis, the breakdown of bone triggers an inflammatory response, which leads to additional destruction of bone. The inflammatory response activates a number of pro-inflammatory cytokines, which tell more white blood cells to get involved. If these cytokines leak into the bloodstream—a very likely event—they can prompt white blood cells throughout the body to react. In TMJ syndrome, the shearing of bone generates large numbers of free radicals, which amplify pain and promote inflammation. All of these disorders are made significantly worse by smoking, which directly exposes oral tissues to large quantities of free radicals and which depletes antioxidants such as vitamin C.

People with periodontitis have a higher than normal risk of suffering heart attacks and strokes; people with any of these conditions commonly have elevated levels of C-reactive protein, a sign of inflammation. In addition, people with diabetes and rheumatoid arthritis—diseases with strong inflammatory components—have a higher risk of developing periodontitis and gingivitis.

Standard Treatment

Conventional dentistry takes a mechanical approach to what is a biological issue. Many dental procedures entail digging into tissues, filing away teeth, and building new structures. For example, the standard treatment for periodontitis in the United States is to clean teeth and then to cut away inflamed tissue. This contrasts with the approach of European dentists, who clean teeth and then allow the tissues to heal over many months. For gingivitis, conventional treatments involve better oral hygiene. TMJ disease is often corrected with a plastic cover over the teeth to separate the upper jaw and the lower jaw.

Dentists know that nonsteroidal anti-inflammatory drugs (NSAIDs) such as ibuprofen can slow the loss of bone in periodontitis. So this question arises: Why not use natural anti-inflammatory nutrients? Unfortunately, the answer is that most dentists are probably less knowledgeable than most physicians about the importance of nutrition in health.

Nutrients That Can Help

For long-term improvements in dental health, it is essential that you start with diet. Nearly everyone is taught that sugar-laden foods feed the bacteria that cause cavities. It is not as well known that sugary foods increase gingival inflammation. Cutting the consumption of sugary foods and soft drinks reduces gingivitis, just as an increased intake of protein and eating less refined carbohydrates, combined with a multivitamin/multimineral supplement, reduces gingivitis.

Vitamin C intake is also important. In one study, researchers found that taking 65 mg of vitamin C daily eased gingival inflammation and bleeding, compared to when subjects received only 5 mg daily. Much larger dosages (605 mg daily), however, led to even greater improvements in gingivitis and bleeding.

Low vitamin C intake is related to larger periodontal "pockets" (spaces around teeth where bone has been lost). Although there are strong parallels between symptoms of gingivitis and periodontitis and the dental ramifications of scurvy (an extreme life-threatening deficiency of vitamin C), there are also major differences. In scurvy, bleeding from the gums is common, and vitamin C can reduce it. Scurvy, however, does not lead to the formation of fibrous scar tissue deep inside the gums, a sign of periodontitis. In addition, lower levels of inflammation are found in periodontitis than in scurvy.

Two other nutrients play key roles in controlling dental inflammation. In an animal study, vitamin E supplements reduced bone loss, very likely because they reduced inflammation. In several small human trials, the topical application of coenzyme Q_{10}, a vitaminlike nutrient, greatly improved periodontitis. To achieve the same benefits, break a soft gelatin capsule of CoQ_{10} (30 to 100 mg), massage its contents into the gums, and swallow the remainder.

Although there has not been any research on the protective roles of omega-3 fish oils or gamma-linolenic acid in dental inflammation, supplements would likely have benefits. In addition, zinc supplements might promote the healing of injured tissues. Calcium and magnesium might help maintain normal bone, and one study has found that glucosamine and chondroitin reduce symptoms of TMJ disease when the joint is affected.

None of this information should negate the value of oral hygiene, but the best hygiene cannot make up for a poor diet and insufficient anti-inflammatory nutrients. Daily flossing and brushing, along with periodic professional cleanings, should be part of the optimal approach to dental health.

What Else Might Help?

Surgery is one of the most common treatments for periodontal disease. It is expensive and painful. Some dentists practice a type of nonsurgical antimicrobial therapy, however, to eliminate infections of the periodontal tissues. The techniques were developed by Paul Keyes, D.D.S., of the National Institutes of Health, and Walter Loesche, D.M.D., Ph.D., a professor emeritus of the University of Michigan School of Dentistry. In a six-and-one-half-year study, Loesche found that patients with periodontal disease were able to preserve 87 percent of their teeth (roughly seven of every eight teeth) originally recommended for extraction or periodontal surgery.

The idea behind Keyes and Loesche's nonsurgical treatment is simple: if bacteria cause periodontal disease, then eliminate the bacteria. Their approaches and those of other dentists (there are variations on the theme) involve spraying antimicrobial compounds (e.g., baking soda, salt water, and Therasol) under the gums. This is easy to do at home with an irrigator (a Waterpik, a ViaJet, or a similar device). Dentists may also prescribe antibiotic drugs or a nonantibiotic antimicrobial drug (e.g., metronidazole) to help reduce bacteria.

This nonsurgical therapy for periodontal disease works, but relatively few periodontists use it because it generates far less revenue compared with surgery. In 2003, my dentist diagnosed a large pocket next to one tooth, evidence of periodontal disease and bone loss. He referred me to a periodontist for surgery, but I was lucky enough to learn of Loesche's protocol, and I found William Helfert, D.D.S., in Mesa, Arizona, who followed the approaches of Keyes and Loesche. The pocket quickly returned to normal depth within several months, and the gums and the tooth remain healthy six years later (as I write this). You can find more information on this approach at two Web sites: www.dent.umich.edu/research/loeschelabs/ and www.mamagums.com, and you can buy most of the supplies you'll need at www.oratec.net. To find a practitioner in your area, look at the partial list of dentists at www.mamagums.com.

Diabetes and Prediabetes

What Is Diabetes?

Diabetes is characterized by chronic elevated levels of blood sugar (glucose) and insulin. Glucose is the body's principal fuel, and insulin helps shuttle it into cells where it is burned for energy. High glucose levels, however, are toxic to the kidneys, and diabetes is associated with a significantly increased risk of heart disease, cancer, kidney failure, blindness, and other diseases. In essence, diabetes accelerates the aging process, so diseases associated with old age occur during middle age.

Causes

Although glucose is blamed for many of the complications of diabetes, growing evidence also points to insulin. For example, people with diabetes who receive large amounts of insulin injections develop vascular disease more rapidly and extensively than do people who use less insulin.

Compelling research suggests that insulin is the oldest, or one of the oldest, hormones in living creatures on Earth. As such, its role is far more fundamental than simply regulating blood sugar levels. It turns on and off various genes and increases the production of body fat and, under different conditions, muscle.

What messes up things? People evolved eating low-carbohydrate foods, which only moderately raise glucose and insulin levels. The consumption of refined carbohydrates and sugars rapidly boosts glucose levels, and the body responds by secreting large amounts of insulin to move the glucose from the blood to cells. After a number of years of dealing with large amounts of glucose, however, cells become resistant to insulin's actions, with the consequence being chronic elevation of both glucose and insulin levels. Insulin resistance is the chief characteristic of diabetes.

Some genetically related groups of people, such as Native Americans, are especially sensitive genetically to insulin resistance and diabetes. But this genetic propensity only means that they develop the disease sooner, rather than later, when exposed to modern Western-style food. Genes aside, the real cause of type 2 diabetes is dietary.

How Common Is Diabetes?

Full-blown type 2 diabetes affects an estimated 24 million Americans, about half of whom have not been officially diagnosed with the disease.

(Type 1 diabetes is an autoimmune disease that is rarely reversible.) As many as 100 million Americans, however, have some form of prediabetes, such as insulin resistance, or Syndrome X. Syndrome X refers to a combination of insulin resistance, high blood pressure, abdominal obesity, and elevated cholesterol and triglycerides. (For more information, see my book *Stop Prediabetes Now.*) Basically, anyone following the typical American diet is consuming foods that increase the risk of insulin resistance, Syndrome X, and diabetes.

The Inflammation Syndrome Connection

High levels of glucose will auto-oxidize—that is, start a chain reaction that produces large amounts of free radicals and "advanced glycation products," both of which damage the body. Free radicals stimulate inflammatory responses and, in this way, people with diabetes develop high levels of inflammation. This situation has been well documented in several studies that have found sharp elevations of CRP and interleukin-6 in people with diabetes. Because of the ability of inflammatory cytokines to stimulate one another, people with diabetes typically have a strong undercurrent of inflammation, which increases the risk of developing other diseases, such as heart disease.

Standard Treatment

Glucose-lowering drugs such as metformin are usually prescribed to people with type 2 diabetes. In severe cases, insulin injections might be added to help lower glucose levels. As you might expect, side effects are common. Metformin interferes with the body's use of B vitamins, and insulin increases body fat, blood pressure, cholesterol levels, and arterial disease. Other drugs also pose problems. Avandia (rosiglitazone maleate) boosts the risk of developing heart disease, and Glucotrol (glipizide), sulfonylureas, and thiazolidinedione cause patients to gain weight.

Nutrients That Can Help

Many supplements can lessen the inflammation in diabetes, but in this case, supplements can be like bailing water in a sinking boat. It is essential that the underlying diet be corrected.

That said, a key objective of supplementation should be to lower glucose levels and improve insulin function, which should in turn reduce inflammation. The chief supplements for improving glucose tolerance and insulin function are alpha-lipoic acid, chromium picolinate, vitamin

D, vitamin C, biotin, and silymarin (an antioxidant extract of the herb milk thistle). If you are taking any drug for controlling glucose, be aware that your medication requirements may decrease.

Alpha-lipoic acid, a natural substance made by the body and found in beef and spinach, is used extensively in Germany to treat diabetic nerve disorders. In daily dosages of 600 mg, it can improve insulin function and lower glucose levels in people with diabetes. It is also a powerful antioxidant.

A lack of chromium results in diabetes-like symptoms. Not surprisingly, therefore, supplements of chromium picolinate, a common form of chromium, have been shown to improve insulin function and lower glucose levels. Sometimes the effects can be significant after several months. In one U.S./Chinese study, diabetic subjects were described as having a "spectacular" improvement after taking 1,000 mcg daily of chromium picolinate for several months.

Vitamins E and C improve glucose tolerance and have the added benefit of lowering levels of CRP and interleukin-6. The effect of these vitamins on easing diabetic complications may be greater than their glucose-lowering properties.

Silymarin can have significant glucose-lowering effects in people with diabetes. An Italian study found major improvements in blood sugar levels and many other symptoms of diabetes after patients took silymarin supplements for one year.

By their nature, antioxidants have anti-inflammatory properties. Some antioxidants also influence the production of cytokines, so they reduce inflammation via another means. Based on insulin's fundamental role in biology, it is likely that the hormone controls the activity of some pro-inflammatory cytokines. It is worthwhile aiming for a fasting glucose level of between 75 and 80 mg/dl and a fasting insulin that is under 7 mcIU/ml.

One of the supplements I often recommend is Nutra-Support Diabetes, which is made by J. R. Carlson Laboratories (www.carlson labs.com). This is a soft-gel multivitamin and multimineral supplement that contains the nutrients and the herbs I mentioned that will help maintain normal blood sugar levels and insulin function.

What Else Might Help?

A person with diabetes must recognize that he or she has a potentially terminal disease, but one that usually can be modified and even reversed through diet. A relatively low-glycemic diet, such as the AI Diet Plan, can moderate the spikes in glucose and insulin that result from eating refined carbohydrates and sugars. Protein will stabilize glucose and insulin levels, and the fiber in vegetables will have a similar effect because it blunts the absorption of carbohydrates.

It would also be worthwhile for people with type 2 diabetes to undergo testing for allergylike food sensitivities. For example, in one case, a person had no significant rise in glucose after eating ice cream but had a several-hundred-point increase in glucose after having Scotch whiskey. A rise or decline of more than 50 points (mg/dl) in one hour is a sign of serious glucose-tolerance problems.

Fatigue and Chronic Fatigue Syndrome

What Are Fatigue and Chronic Fatigue Syndrome?

Fatigue is the most common complaint that physicians hear from their patients, and it is the principal reason behind one of every five visits to internists and family physicians. The term is generally used to describe persistent feelings of tiredness and low energy levels. In contrast, chronic fatigue syndrome (CFS) refers to a debilitating fatigue that lasts for six months or longer. CFS symptoms tend to include impaired concentration and short-term memory, sore throat, tender lymph nodes, muscle pain, and a significant increase in fatigue following exertion. Psychological issues, particularly depression, are also a common symptom of CFS.

Causes

Feelings of chronic fatigue can be a symptom of many different diseases, including heart failure and cancer. Most people who feel chronically fatigued at home and at work, however, are usually prediabetic, diabetic, or sleep deprived. The reason is that elevated blood sugar levels inhibit brain chemicals known as orexins, which are needed for alertness; feeling sleepy shortly after lunch or dinner is often a sign of abnormally high blood sugar. At the same time, the body secretes a variety of pro-inflammatory cytokines, including interleukin-6 and C-reactive protein, which may contribute to feelings of fatigue. In contrast, CFS often follows flulike symptoms, infection with the Epstein-Barr virus (which also causes mononucleosis), or some sort of toxic chemical exposure (such as to a large amount of pesticides). It is possible that in some people, the virus or the toxic exposure causes mutations in mitochondria, the energy factories of cells.

How Common Are Fatigue and Chronic Fatigue Syndrome?

An estimated 1 million Americans have CFS, but, according to the Centers for Disease Control and Prevention, tens of millions of other people have comparable feelings of fatigue, but their symptoms do not meet the strict definition of CFS.

The Inflammation Syndrome Connection

Psychological and physical stresses increase the secretion of pro-inflammatory substances, including interleukin-1 beta, interleukin-6, and C-reactive protein. A report published in the January 2009 *Archives of General Psychiatry* noted that people who had been emotionally and sexually abused in childhood were six times more likely to have CFS as adults, compared with people who did not experience those types of maltreatment. Stress increases the production of pro-inflammatory cytokines.

Standard Treatment

Conventional medical treatments are geared toward easing symptoms and improving physical functioning. Physical therapy may be helpful. Treatments tend to be individualized.

Nutrients That Can Help

Because prediabetes or type 2 diabetes may be the cause of persistent feelings of fatigue, a protein-rich, low-carbohydrate diet (such as the AI Diet Plan) is often helpful in lowering and stabilizing blood sugar levels. Several nutrients involved in mitochondrial chemical reactions are likely to be helpful. These nutrients include CoQ_{10}, L-carnitine or acetyl-L-carnitine, alpha-lipoic acid, and ribose. Some preliminary research suggests that quercetin, an antioxidant, stimulates the breakdown of food to energy and increases the number of mitochondria.

What Else Might Help?

To help build muscle and to increase the numbers of mitochondria in cells, it is important to begin a resistance-exercise program. Because fatigue may initially be exacerbated, begin the program slowly and build up exercise tolerance. A personal trainer can help, but be sure to advise him or her of your limitations. Alternatively, using hand weights and walking are good starting points. In addition, mitochondrial nutrients (see the previous paragraph) might help in terms of developing tolerance. A multi–amino acid supplement or a branched-chain amino acid supplement might also help build muscle. As muscle mass is augmented, the number of mitochondria per cell will also increase,

Mononucleosis, caused by the Epstein-Barr virus, can infect people of any age and can rapidly progress to CFS. To reduce the risk of such a progression, find a nutritionally oriented physician (M.D. or N.D.) to administer two weekly 50-gram intravenous vitamin C infusions for several months. Intravenous Vitamin C works better when used soon after the diagnosis of mononucleosis. The cost for each infusion should be around $100. If this seems high, it is an inexpensive alternative to feeling fatigued for years to come.

Fibromyalgia

What Is Fibromyalgia?

Fibromyalgia is characterized by feelings of pain "all over" and an exacerbation of pain from simple touch. Extreme fatigue is also common, but unlike chronic fatigue syndrome, pain is the principal symptom. Other symptoms include depression, moodiness, dry eyes and skin, and anxiety. Fibromyalgia affects nine times more women than men, and it is frequently associated with sleep problems, irritable bowel syndrome, headaches, facial pain, and sensitivity to odors and noises.

Causes

Most articles on fibromyalgia that are published by conventional medical organizations, such as the Mayo Clinic, state that no one knows what causes the disease; however, infections, injuries in the spinal area, and sleep problems may predispose some people to develop fibromyalgia.

How Common Is Fibromyalgia?

Fibromyalgia is estimated to affect 3 to 8 million Americans.

The Inflammation Syndrome Connection

Doctors disagree on the role of inflammation in fibromyalgia. Many believe that inflammation is not part of the disorder. A study published in the March–April 2007 issue of *Clinical and Experimental Rheumatology*, however, clearly showed that several promoters of inflammation—specifically, tumor necrosis factor alpha, interleukin-8, and interleukin-10—were elevated and directly related to symptoms in patients with fibromyalgia.

Standard Treatment

Conventional treatments include an assortment of drugs, such as analgesics, antidepressants, and muscle relaxants. It is very likely that side effects from these drugs contribute to the general feelings of malaise. The drug Lyrica (pregabalin) is heavily advertised for the treatment of fibromyalgia, but it is potentially addictive.

Nutrients That Can Help

Many symptoms of fibromyalgia are suggestive of nutritional deficiencies, which are usually overlooked. For example, dry skin and eyes can be signs of a deficiency of essential fatty acids, such as EPA, DHA, and GLA. These fatty acids may also reduce pain. The B-complex vitamins have an analgesic benefit, and they may alleviate the moodiness, depression, and anxiety of many patients. Vitamin D also has analgesic and mood-lifting benefits.

Recently, researchers reported that taking two 500-mg supplements daily of acetyl-L-carnitine led to improvements in depression and musculoskeletal pain in fibromyalgia patients. Intramuscular injections of acetyl-L-carnitine also helped. Another study, published in *Clinical Biochemistry* in 2009, suggested that supplemental CoQ_{10} might be helpful as well.

What Else Might Help?

A study at the Mayo Clinic found that acupuncture led to a significant amelioration of fibromyalgia symptoms. Stress-reduction activities, such as meditation and yoga, might also be helpful.

Gastritis, Ulcers, and Stomach Cancer

What Are Gastritis, Ulcers, and Stomach Cancer?

Gastritis refers to an inflammation of the stomach wall, as well as of the uppermost part of the small intestine, the duodenum. An ulcer, such as a peptic ulcer, is a lesion on the wall of the stomach. The most serious ulcers form deep craters or bleed. Gastric cancer is a growth of abnormal cells on the stomach wall. Sometimes, but not always, gastritis will evolve into an ulcer, and both conditions increase the risk of gastric cancer.

Causes

For many years, physicians believed that gastritis was the result of excess stomach acid, and drug treatments were designed to reduce the secretion of gastric juices or to make them more alkaline. In 1983, researchers identified a type of bacterium, *Helicobacter pylori*, in the stomach, and in the 1990s it was recognized as the leading cause of gastritis, ulcers, and stomach cancer. Conventional treatment now focuses on antibiotics and drugs that reduce the secretion of gastric juices.

There is a wrinkle to this story, however. With the successful use of antibiotics in eradicating *H. pylori* infections, a new leading cause of gastritis and ulcers has emerged: nonsteroidal anti-inflammatory drugs (NSAIDs), such as aspirin, ibuprofen, and coxibs. All NSAIDs, including the so-called Cox-2 selective drugs, disrupt the activity of cyclooxygenase-1 (Cox-1), an enzyme that is essential for fatty acid production and for maintaining the health of the stomach wall.

How Common Are Gastritis, Ulcers, and Stomach Cancer?

Gastritis affects roughly 5 million Americans. Although stomach cancer does not garner many headlines, it is the second most common fatal cancer in the world, and in most countries the five-year survival rates are less than 20 percent. Chronic *H. pylori* infections boost the risk of developing stomach cancer by up to 80 percent.

The Inflammation Syndrome Connection

H. pylori irritates the stomach wall, but the immune response to this infection may wreak most of the damage. *H. pylori* leads to greater production of a pro-inflammatory cytokine, interleukin-1 beta, which has been specifically linked to the development of stomach cancer, according to an article in the November 4, 2008, issue of *Cancer Cell*. In addition, white blood cells are mobilized to the site of the infection, where they release free radicals and pro-inflammatory eicosanoids such as prostaglandin E_2. *H. pylori* is often highly resistant to this immune response, which can inflame the stomach wall and may eventually lead to an ulcer. Free radicals damage the DNA in stomach wall cells, increasing the chance of mutations, some of which could seed cancers.

The high levels of free radicals in the stomach rapidly deplete antioxidant levels in gastric juices and the stomach wall, and numerous studies have found that gastritis and gastric ulcers are associated with low levels of vitamins E and C and beta-carotene. The situation is made worse when people consume relatively few fruits and vegetables, the principal dietary sources of antioxidants. In a Scottish study, researchers reported that *H. pylori* infection interfered with the body's utilization of vitamin C. When people infected with *H. pylori* ate few fruits and vegetables, their vitamin C levels dropped to one-third less than normal. Another study, conducted at the University of Auckland, New Zealand, found that people with *H. pylori* infections had only one-fifteenth the vitamin C in their gastric acid, compared with healthy subjects. Similar research has found that *H. pylori* compromises levels of vitamin E and the carotenoids, a situation that increases the risk of getting nearly every disease.

Standard Treatment

Antacids and drugs that alter the osmotic flow are commonly prescribed for gastritis and ulcers. A course of antibiotics is typically prescribed for people with gastritis or ulcers caused by *H. pylori* bacteria. Gastric cancer is treated with surgery or radiation.

Nutrients That Can Help

An impressive body of research, including clinical trials, has found that antioxidants strongly influence whether an *H. pylori* infection leads to gastritis, ulcers, or stomach cancer. Antioxidants can sometimes eliminate an *H. pylori* infection, although it is probably more judicious to use them in conjunction with antibiotics.

The most dramatic study investigated both antioxidant supplements and antibiotic therapy. Pelayo Correa, M.D., of Louisiana State University, New Orleans, asked 631 people with precancerous changes in their stomach-wall cells to take 30 mg of beta-carotene (50,000 IU) or 2 grams of vitamin C daily, a combination of both antioxidants, or a placebo for six years. Some of the subjects also underwent standard two-week antibiotic treatment for *H. pylori*, and others received both antioxidants and antibiotics. Changes to the gut were examined through endoscopy or biopsy after three and six years.

Correa found that three treatments—beta-carotene, vitamin C, and antibiotics—resulted in significant reversals of the precancerous stomach cells. In the treatment of nonmetaplastic atrophy, one type of precancerous condition, people receiving beta-carotene, vitamin C, or antibiotics were about five times more likely to improve than were those receiving no treatment. Similarly, people with intestinal metaplasia, another type of precancerous condition, were almost 3½ times more likely to improve. In both cases, the benefits of beta-carotene edged out vitamin C, and vitamin C edged out antibiotics. A combination of beta-carotene and vitamin C provided no additional benefits; however, 15 percent of the people taking antioxidants alone (no antibiotics) were cured of their *H. pylori* infection.

Two other studies have found that vitamin C supplements are beneficial. In a small trial sponsored by the World Health Organization, researchers gave 5 grams of vitamin C daily for four weeks to thirty-two people with chronic gastritis and *H. pylori* infections. The supplements eradicated *H. pylori* infections in 30 percent of the patients. In Italy, fifty-eight patients were treated with antibiotics, followed by either 500 mg of vitamin C daily for six months or no further treatment at all. Precancerous gastric cells were reversed in about a third of the patients taking vitamin C. In contrast, only one patient (technically, 3.4 percent) from the other group improved.

What Else Might Help?

Other antioxidants may also offer protection against *H. pylori* infections and their consequential damage to the stomach. Among these are the herb Ginkgo biloba and garlic. Lycopene, a carotenoid that gives tomatoes their red color, has been associated with a relatively low risk of developing stomach cancer, although this association does not directly prove prevention. In addition, animal experiments suggest that food allergies might also irritate the stomach and lead to gastritis and ulcers.

An estimated 30 percent of people over age sixty-five suffer from atrophic gastritis, a chronic inflammation of the stomach associated with a wasting away of stomach tissues. The condition sharply increases the likelihood of vitamin B_{12} deficiency, which is significant because low levels of these vitamins can cause senile symptoms. It is important to keep in mind that the risk of atrophic gastritis does not suddenly appear at a certain age, but that it is a consequence of more subtle changes to stomach tissue and function. Although research in this area has focused on vitamin B_{12}, it is likely that atrophic gastritis and other forms of gastritis interfere with the absorption of many other nutrients. In addition, antiulcer drugs that inhibit the secretion of gastric juices could conceivably increase the long-term risk of developing atrophic gastritis.

Gastritis is often associated with frequent heartburn and its more severe form, gastric reflux. Prilosec, Prevacid, Nexium, and other proton-pump inhibitor drugs lower levels of vitamins C and B_{12}. L-arginine may help with gastric reflux, and melatonin may also be of benefit. In addition, eating smaller portions and avoiding food allergens (often undiagnosed) can help.

Hepatitis

What Is Hepatitis?

Hepatitis literally means "liver inflammation." It is usually, though not always, caused by a viral infection. Symptoms of acute hepatitis, a disease that generally lasts fewer than six months, tend to appear suddenly and include fever, nausea, vomiting, and a general feeling of being ill. Many cases of acute hepatitis evolve into chronic low-grade liver infections.

Sometimes people with chronic hepatitis may be asymptomatic, and at other times they may experience extreme fatigue and loss of appetite. In both acute and chronic hepatitis, liver enzymes become elevated—one sign of liver disease. Noninfectious hepatitis may result from drug or alcohol abuse. Often, the stress of hepatitis reduces levels of glutathione, one of the body's principal antioxidants, which is made in the liver. The viral and inflammatory stresses, combined with low glutathione levels, compromise liver function and may lead to cirrhosis or liver failure.

Causes

Viral hepatitis is caused by one of several viruses that attack the liver. The various types of hepatitis are referred to by a letter, as in hepatitis A or hepatitis B. Transmission of the different viruses occurs in a variety of ways. For example, hepatitis A is usually transmitted through fecal contamination of food, whereas hepatitis B is typically transmitted through sexual contact or shared needles. Hepatitis C is passed through the blood, such as via shared needles or through pre-1991 blood transfusions. There are still other forms of hepatitis. One laboratory indication of hepatitis infection is an elevation in liver enzyme levels.

How Common Is Hepatitis?

Hepatitis C has received the lion's share of attention in recent years, and an estimated 4 million Americans have chronic hepatitis C infections. Many people have the disease without symptoms, and it may take decades for chronic hepatitis to become clinically apparent. Approximately 10,000 Americans die each year as a result of hepatitis C infections.

The Inflammation Syndrome Connection

Inflammation is the body's normal response to infection. But in chronic infection, the sustained immune activity may cause as much damage as, if not more than, the infection itself. From a biological standpoint, inflammation is very costly—stressful—to an organ. The liver is the body's largest organ, and it functions as a chemical processing plant, building needed molecules and breaking down toxins. This is a complex and diverse job, and the stress of a liver-specific infection is tantamount to a worker strike. When tissue damage and scarring become extensive, cirrhosis or liver failure may be the end result. Hepatitis results in more cases of liver failure than any other cause.

Standard Treatment

The most common pharmaceutical treatment is interferon, a synthetic version of a natural immune compound. Interferon is expensive, however, and frequently causes flulike symptoms that last for months.

Nutrients That Can Help

Burton M. Berkson, M.D., Ph.D., of Las Cruces, New Mexico, has found that a combination of three liver-supporting nutrients can control and reduce symptoms of hepatitis C. These nutrients are alpha-lipoic acid (discussed in chapter 11); selenium (also discussed in chapter 11); and silymarin, an extract of the herb milk thistle.

In the 1970s and 1980s, Berkson used large doses of alpha-lipoic acid to treat *Amanita* mushroom poisoning, which often precipitates liver failure and death. Alpha-lipoic acid boosts the liver's production of glutathione, which aids the breakdown of *Amanita* toxins and promotes the synthesis of new liver cells. Similarly, selenium is needed for the liver to make several glutathione peroxidase compounds, all potent antioxidants. The herb milk thistle has been used for thousands of years as a liver tonic, and its silymarin extract is now recognized as a powerful antioxidant.

As with *Amanita* toxins (and many other toxic substances), the liver carries the burden of breaking down the poisons. Berkson has found that the combination of alpha-lipoic acid (600 mg daily), selenium (400 mcg daily), and silymarin (900 mg daily) is especially effective in lowering liver enzymes and restoring liver function.

What Else Might Help?

If you received a blood transfusion before 1991, when blood banks began testing for hepatitis C, it might be worthwhile for you to be tested. Even if the test provides bad news, it enables you to take steps to deal with the infection, instead of allowing it to quietly run its destructive course.

Infections

What Are Infections?

Infections result from an attack on the body by pathogenic (disease-causing) bacteria, viruses, parasites, or prions. There are many ways to group infections, but for our purposes it is best to view them as either acute or chronic. Acute infections occur suddenly, such as in the case of colds and flus, followed by recovery. Chronic infections such as hepatitis or HIV/AIDS last many years and may be the ultimate cause of death. That said, acute infections can be very dangerous in themselves—the flu kills approximately 20,000 Americans each year.

Causes

Most pathogens need a warm body to flourish. When they enter the body, typically through the mouth or the nose and sometimes via the blood (such as through a cut or a transfusion), they trigger an immune response designed to destroy bacteria or virus-infected cells. Yet many viruses and parasites can evade the immune response. A person's ability to resist infection, as well as to moderate symptoms of the infection, relates in large part to the health and efficiency of the immune system. The state of one's nutrition has a direct bearing on immune efficiency.

How Common Are Infections?

Everyone contracts an infection from time to time, whether it's a cold or an infected cut. Worldwide, infections have always been and are still the leading cause of death. If all of the infection-caused deaths in the United States were combined, they would be the third leading cause of death there, after cancer and heart disease.

The Inflammation Syndrome Connection

The immune system's inflammatory response is designed to kill pathogens. In colds, flus, and other acute infections, inflammation accounts for many of the symptoms, such as rhinitis, tenderness, and aches and pains. The consequence of this inflammation may last beyond the actual infection. As one example, Robert Cathcart III, M.D., of Los Altos, California, has pointed out that the stress of a cold or a flu can lead to symptoms of an extreme vitamin C deficiency. That lack of vitamin C limits the body's ability to "clean up" excess free radicals produced by the immune system. These unquenched free radicals can cause considerable wear and tear on the body.

In many respects chronic infections, whether low-grade (such as parasitic infections) or more serious infections (such as HIV/AIDS), are more insidious. They force the immune system to remain at a heightened state of stressful activity, draining many of the body's nutritional and biochemical reserves. For example, people with HIV/AIDS often experience chronic diarrhea, which is likely the result of inflammatory bowel disease. The diarrhea limits absorption of essential nutrients, and high levels of vitamins and mineral supplements may be needed to achieve normal blood values. A similar situation is true of sepsis, in which the immune response can be as deadly as the infection itself.

Standard Treatment

Most over-the-counter treatments relieve symptoms but often with undesirable side effects. For example, antihistamines may reduce nasal congestion, but they cause drowsiness and, long term, they may increase the risk of cancer. Antibiotics can kill many types of pathogenic bacteria, but they disrupt some aspects of immunity and cause gastric disturbances. Some antiviral drugs reduce flu symptoms but so far not to the extent of vitamin C or N-acetylcysteine (NAC). More powerful antiviral drugs can cause genetic damage.

Nutrients That Can Help

In general, the supplements that reduce symptoms of colds and flus can, in higher dosages, reduce symptoms and extend the life span in people with much more serious infections, such as HIV/AIDS. These nutrients do not have direct antiviral activity. Rather, they enhance the immune system's ability to confront the infection, as well as to prevent nutritional deficiencies that further compromise health.

Beginning in the 1970s, Robert Cathcart III, M.D., has used large amounts of vitamin C, orally and at times intravenously, to treat patients with a variety of infections, including colds, flus, mononucleosis, hepatitis, and HIV/AIDS. Sometimes the dosages are truly massive, such as 100 grams or more daily. Cathcart found that people usually can tolerate large oral amounts of vitamin C without developing diarrhea when they are ill. As people recover, such large dosages of vitamin C become excessive and cause diarrhea, a sign that the dosage should be reduced. Huge dosages of vitamin C may not always be necessary, though. In a review of twenty-one studies on vitamin C and the common cold, Harri Hemila, Ph.D., a professor at the University of Helsinki, Finland, found that 2 to 6 grams of vitamin C daily reduced the duration and severity of symptoms by about a third.

NAC is a potent antioxidant that, despite an unpleasant sulfur odor, has a significant effect on the symptoms and the course of infections. It may in fact be superior to vitamin C. In a study of 262 elderly people, supplements of 600 mg of NAC daily reduced the occurrence of flu symptoms by two-thirds, and many people with laboratory-confirmed flu infections had no symptoms at all. In addition, researchers at Stanford University have reported that high dosages of NAC significantly extend the life expectancy of AIDS patients.

NAC can also help people with sepsis and septic shock. Sepsis, an infection of the blood, often pushes hospitalized patients to a life-or-death situation—not because of a pathogen but from an overwhelming immune response to the infection. Researchers reported in the journal *Chest* that NAC reduced recovery times in patients with septic shock. NAC works in part by boosting glutathione, the most powerful of the body's own antioxidants. Selenium, part of the antioxidant enzyme glutathione peroxidase, increases survival among patients who have a condition that has similarities to sepsis, severe system inflammatory response syndrome.

What Else Might Help?

To reduce the risk of contracting colds and flus, it is important to exercise caution when interacting with infected people. For example, wash your hands after touching a person (or touching objects the person has recently touched) who has such an infection. To reduce your risk of contracting HIV and certain types of hepatitis, avoid unprotected sexual contact or other exchanges of body fluids, such as through the use of unsterilized syringes.

Supplements of the herb echinacea stimulate immunity and appear to boost resistance to infections. It is possible that, as with NAC, echinacea does not protect against infections so much as it enhances immunity and renders symptoms negligible. Similarly, one clinical study unexpectedly found that people taking vitamin E supplements had 30 percent fewer colds. Lozenges containing zinc, a mineral needed for immunity, can significantly reduce cold and flu symptoms in many people, although the clinical findings have been mixed. The list of nutrients can go on, but it is important to remember that any deficiency impairs many aspects of health, including the degree of symptoms during an infection.

In children, food allergies can increase the risk of ear infections. Allergies lead to fluid retention in the ears (which do not drain as well in infants and children as they do in adults), forming a breeding ground for bacteria. Eliminating the most likely food allergens, such as dairy and wheat products, can cut down on the risk of ear infections.

Reduce the inflammatory stress caused by both acute and chronic infections. By doing so, you lessen the long-term damage—wear and tear, if you wish—from activated immune cells acting against their host.

Irritable Bowel Syndrome

What Is Irritable Bowel Syndrome?

Ulcerative colitis and Crohn's disease are the two types of irritable bowel syndrome (IBS). Both ulcerative colitis and Crohn's disease have similarities, and often it is difficult to distinguish between the two. As a general rule, ulcerative colitis is an inflammation limited to the wall of the colon (bowel). Its symptoms include abdominal cramps, fever, and bloody diarrhea. Similar symptoms, generally affecting the ileum (a portion of the small intestine) and without blood in the stools, are generally suggestive of Crohn's disease.

Causes

Officially, medicine does not know the cause of ulcerative colitis and Crohn's disease. The fact that IBS affects the digestive tract, however, strongly points to an interaction with food.

How Common Is Irritable Bowel Syndrome?

An estimated 500,000 to 1 million Americans have either ulcerative colitis or Crohn's disease. People of Jewish descent are more likely than Gentiles to develop IBS.

The Inflammation Syndrome Connection

The abdominal cramps, which may come on suddenly, are spasmodic responses to an irritant. Various pro-inflammatory cytokines are elevated in people with IBS. The combination can lead to a "leaky gut" in which undigested food proteins move into the blood, causing a broader immune response.

Standard Treatment

A variety of drugs, including corticosteroids, may be prescribed for IBS. The role of diet is often ignored.

Nutrients That Can Help

It should come as no surprise that anti-inflammatory omega-3 fatty acids are helpful in relieving IBS. In a study published in the *New England Journal of Medicine*, researchers described how they gave 500-mg fish oil capsules or placebos daily to thirty-nine patients with Crohn's disease for one year. Only 28 percent of the people taking fish oil capsules had relapses of Crohn's disease, whereas almost two-thirds of those taking placebos experienced relapses. A much higher dose—7 to 15 grams daily—might prove more helpful.

Low levels of antioxidants might also hinder the body's ability to ease the inflammation. Canadian researchers have reported that people with Crohn's disease have elevated levels of "oxidative stress," a sign of inadequate antioxidants—even when symptoms are controlled by medication. For example, compared with healthy subjects, people with Crohn's disease had low selenium levels.

What Else Might Help?

It is essential that a person with IBS investigate the possibility of food sensitivities. The most likely dietary culprits are gluten-containing foods (wheat, rye, barley, and nearly every type of processed food) and dairy products. Eliminating these foods should improve symptoms within one to two weeks, if they were a cause of IBS.

One recent report by French researchers found that half of a group of 171 patients with Crohn's disease had elevated levels of homocysteine, a sign of folic acid and vitamin B_{12} deficiency. This does not necessarily mean that these B-vitamin deficiencies cause Crohn's disease, although they could be involved. Rather, the deficiencies may be a consequence of Crohn's disease that, over many years, could increase the risk of heart disease or stroke.

A recent study by physicians at the Yale University School of Medicine, published in *Phytomedicine*, found that the herb wormwood (*Artemisia absinthium*) significantly reduced symptoms of Crohn's disease. Forty patients were given either 750 mg of the SedaCrohn brand of wormwood or placebos twice daily for ten weeks. After eight weeks, thirteen (65 percent) of the twenty patients taking wormwood had an almost full remission of symptoms. As a result, they were able to reduce their use of corticosteroid drugs. Most of the patients taking placebos had a worsening of their symptoms.

Lupus Erythematosus

What Is Lupus Erythematosus?

Lupus erythematosus is an autoimmune disease, meaning that the inflammation-causing immune cells attack the body's own tissues. It can affect different parts of the body, such as the skin, joints, kidneys, lungs, and cardiovascular system, and can cause a wide variety of symptoms. Some cases are very mild, whereas others may be disabling or fatal. Ninety percent of people with lupus experience inflammation of their connective tissue, with symptoms often similar to rheumatoid arthritis, another autoimmune disease. Other common symptoms include rashes, sensitivity to sunlight, and kidney disorders.

Causes

No one really understands the cause or causes of lupus. Fever is common at its onset, suggesting that a bacterial or viral infection initiates the immune response (although inadequate vitamin B_1 may also cause fever). The hormone estrogen may influence lupus because it is most often diagnosed in women between their late teens and thirties; however, a hormonal link is tempered by the fact that estrogen therapies have not been useful as a treatment. It is conceivable that a woman's immune system is simply biologically different in some ways from that of a man.

How Common Is Lupus Erythematosus?

Lupus affects approximately 1.6 million people in the United States, ten times as many women as men.

The Inflammation Syndrome Connection

As with other inflammatory diseases, particularly rheumatoid arthritis and multiple sclerosis, some factor or event turns immune cells against their host. Periods of remission are common, although lupus symptoms and tissue damage typically become worse with time.

Standard Treatment

Conventional treatments are intended to reduce inflammation and include corticosteroids, as well as a variety of other immune-suppressing medications.

Nutrients That Can Help

As many as three of every four people with lupus experience flare-ups when exposed to sunlight. Limiting exposure to sunlight increases the risk of people developing vitamin D deficiency, which is unfortunate because the vitamin may help reduce symptoms of lupus through its role as an immune-modulating hormone. The solution is to take vitamin D supplements. Ideally, patients should ask their physicians to specifically measure their blood levels of "25 (OH) vitamin D," then supplement as needed to achieve normal levels. If you cannot get a blood test for vitamin D, it's safe to take 2,000 IU daily of vitamin D_3. Low levels of vitamin D are common in other types of autoimmune diseases, such as rheumatoid arthritis and multiple sclerosis.

Some research also suggests that curcumin, an extract from the spice turmeric, might help alleviate lupus symptoms. In addition, the hormone dehydroepiandrosterone (DHEA) might help.

Omega-3 fatty acids and vitamin E may help in controlling lupus. The evidence is more derivative than direct, based on the anti-inflammatory nature of these nutrients. A clinical trial published in *Arthritis and Rheumatism* found that large dosages of DHEA may be beneficial. Supplements, which are available at health food stores, lessened the frequency of flare-ups; however, DHEA should be used under a physician's guidance.

One intriguing European study, published in *Phytotherapy Research,* found that supplements of flavonoid-containing Pycnogenol significantly reduced markers of inflammation and disease activity in patients with lupus. Patients taking corticosteroids to suppress inflammatory symptoms benefited from greater reductions in symptoms after adding 120 mg daily of Pycnogenol, and they also experienced decreases in their sedimentation rate, a general indicator of inflammation. It is possible that grape-seed extract and other flavonoids might be beneficial as well.

What Else Might Help?

Although there is no clinical evidence to document its usefulness, it might be worthwhile to adopt (at least for a few weeks) a Paleolithic-style diet similar to the AI Diet Plan, as well as eliminating nightshade plants (such as tomatoes, potatoes, peppers, and eggplants). Such a diet provides high-quality protein and antioxidant-rich vegetables and fruit. At the same time, this diet eliminates calorie-dense carbohydrates, highly refined cooking oils, and trans-fatty acids.

In addition, it might be helpful to take vitamin D supplements (400 to 800 IU daily). Researchers at the University of Utrecht, Netherlands, reported that vitamin D deficiency is common among patients with lupus, either because they spend little time in the sun or because of how some medications interfere with the vitamin.

Multiple Sclerosis

What Is Multiple Sclerosis?

Multiple sclerosis (MS) is generally considered an autoimmune disease, in which immune cells attack the myelin sheaths wrapped around nerve fibers. *Sclerosis* is the medical term for "lesion," and in MS multiple scarlike lesions form on the myelin, which is akin to the plastic insulation surrounding electrical wires. When the myelin becomes inflamed, it literally begins to fray, short-circuiting nerve signals and leading to the disease's physical and neurological symptoms.

Different MS symptoms are related to the location of specific nerve damage. They can take the form of extreme fatigue, weakness, a lack of balance, difficulty walking, double vision, speech problems, and depression.

Causes

Officially, there is no known cause of MS; however, it is clearly related to an immune response that goes seriously awry. This immune reaction might be triggered by allergylike sensitivities, a viral attack, a physical injury, or any number of other insults, but the sustained damage appears to be related to the immune system. Although people with MS may have periods of remission, symptoms typically become worse—and crippling—over the years. On average, the life expectancy of people with MS is about a fourth less than that of people without the disease.

How Common Is Multiple Sclerosis?

MS affects an estimated 400,000 Americans and about 2.5 million people worldwide. For reasons that remain mysterious, it strikes more women than men, most often between ages twenty and forty, and people of northern European descent (in contrast to Asians and Africans). According to a study at the University of California, San Francisco, the stress of daily hassles and major life events can exacerbate MS symptoms.

MS researchers have long recognized that the incidence of MS generally increases farther north and south from the equator, correlating to less sunlight. Sunlight activates the body's production of vitamin D, and people living farther from the equator would, over the course of a year, make less vitamin D. This relationship doesn't confirm that a lack of vitamin D increases the risk of contracting MS, but there are other tantalizing data. According to a report by C. E. Hayes, Ph.D., and his colleagues at the University of Wisconsin, Madison, vitamin D can prevent experimental autoimmune encephalomyelitis, the mouse version of human MS.

The Inflammation Syndrome Connection

In autoimmune diseases, most tissue damage is caused by immune cells, rather than by the event (if it is even identifiable) that triggered the immune response. For example, a form of the herpes virus known as *human herpes virus 6* seems to promote MS flare-ups, although most people harbor the virus without developing the disease.

What causes the immune overreactivity? It often seems to be related to a lack of anti-inflammatory nutrients in the diet. The modern diet, with a lopsided intake of fats, particularly highly refined fats and oils, may set the stage for MS in genetically susceptible people.

Although the prevalence of MS increases at extreme northern and southern latitudes, people living along the coast of Norway and throughout Japan have a relatively low incidence of MS. These populations eat large amounts of fish, which are rich in anti-inflammatory omega-3 fatty acids.

Standard Treatment

Medications include short-term use of corticosteroids to suppress immune activity, as well as interferon.

Nutrients That Can Help

Physicians at Trondheim University Hospital, Norway, have reported that 0.9 gram daily of omega-3 fish oil supplements significantly reduced MS symptoms in sixteen patients. In general, gamma-linolenic acid, found in borage seed oil, evening primrose oil, and olive oil, enhances the anti-inflammatory effects of omega-3 fatty acids, so a combination of supplements might be ideal.

The perplexing increase in MS in extreme northern and southern regions might be explained by inadequate vitamin D. The body makes vitamin D when exposed to sunlight, but extreme latitudes have long winters and relatively few daylight hours. Research by Colleen E. Hayes, Ph.D., a biochemist at the University of Wisconsin, Madison, has shown that vitamin D suppresses the autoimmune reaction underlying MS. In experiments with laboratory mice, Hayes found that vitamin D raised levels of two anti-inflammatory compounds (interleukin-4 and transforming growth factor beta-1) and stopped the progression of the animals' version of MS.

Brief exposures to sunlight (fifteen to thirty minutes daily) stimulate the body's production of vitamin D, and people living or working in sunny climates may produce more than 10,000 IU daily. According to Hayes, a very high dose—4,000 IU daily—may be required to achieve normal levels of the vitamin among people who do not receive sunlight.

What Else Might Help?

Several other nutrients might reduce MS symptoms. Antioxidants such as vitamin E, flavonoids, and alpha-lipoic acid might ease inflammation.

Vitamin B_{12} might also be of value. Several years ago E. H. Reynolds, M.D., of King's College Hospital, London, found that MS patients were almost always deficient in vitamin B_{12}, which is needed for normal nerve function. Japanese researchers gave MS patients huge dosages of vitamin B_{12} (60 mg, not mcg, daily) for six months. Their visual and auditory symptoms improved, but muscle function did not.

Because dietary fats have been so skewed by refining and processing, it might be worthwhile to adopt a Paleolithic-style diet similar to the one described in this book. Emphasizing anti-inflammatory fats and studiously avoiding pro-inflammatory trans-fatty acids might have benefits.

Overweight and Obesity

What Are Overweight and Obesity?

By clinical definition, a person is obese when an individual is thirty or more pounds over his or her ideal weight. Simply being overweight is characterized by being a few pounds to up to thirty pounds over his or her ideal weight. Of course, a well-trained muscular person might be incorrectly considered overweight because muscle tissue is more dense and heavy than fat tissue. Therefore, accurate assessments should calculate fat-to-muscle or hip-to-waist ratios. From a practical standpoint, a look in the mirror can make much of the testing unnecessary. Most people who are overweight or obese know that they are, although they might want to deny the obvious.

Causes

Overweight and obesity usually are diseases of overeating, although metabolic factors affect some people. The traditional view is that people gain weight when they consume more calories than they burn. This is partly true because many people are not as physically active as their ancestors were, but it fails to explain everything.

Often ignored is that diet can serve to exacerbate or moderate a preexisting metabolic disorder. In addition, the source of calories is at least as important as the overall quantity of calories. That is because protein is far less likely than carbohydrate to be stored as fat. In general, high-sugar and high-carbohydrate foods trigger a stronger insulin response, compared with protein-rich foods, and insulin helps promote the accumulation of body fat. High-sugar and high-carbohydrate foods also tend to be short on fiber, protein, omega-3 fatty acids, and vitamins and minerals that either buffer the absorption of carbohydrates or aid in the body's metabolism of them.

Several animal studies have found that certain dietary fats are more likely than others to become body fat. For example, some research shows that consumption of monounsaturated fat results in less body fat than does saturated fat, even when both provide the same number of calories. Similarly, evidence suggests that consumption of omega-3 fatty acids, calorie for calorie, might result in relatively less body fat.

Trans fats, found in hydrogenated oils and interesterified fats, interfere with the normal metabolism of omega-3 and omega-6 fats and, according to studies in primates, promote the formation of belly fat. Trans fats are also pro-inflammatory. In addition, high-fructose corn syrup is more "lipogenic" than regular sugar (sucrose), meaning that it is especially good at being converted to fat in the body. Trans fats and high-fructose corn syrup are found in many packaged foods. They are most easily avoided if you consume fresh foods. I discuss these food ingredients and ways to avoid them in more detail in my book *Stop Prediabetes Now*.

How Common Are Overweight and Obesity?

The prevalence of obesity and overweight have, without exaggeration, skyrocketed in recent years. In 2001, David Satcher, M.D., then the surgeon general of the United States, described it as an "epidemic." He predicted that the health consequences of overweight and obesity would soon overtake the effects of tobacco. Three of every four American adults are now overweight, and one-half of overweight people are actually obese. The number of overweight children ranges from approximately one in five to one in three.

These increases in weight result largely from the increased consumption of junk foods that consist chiefly of refined sugars, carbohydrates, and fats. A major source of dietary sugar is soft drinks, which the consumer-oriented Center for Science in the Public Interest has described as "liquid candy." A 64-ounce bottle of any calorically sweetened (in contrast to artificially sweetened) soft drink contains approximately ½ cup of sugar! Children have essentially been weaned on soft drinks and calorie-dense fast-food restaurant fare. "Super-size" meals lead to super-size children and adults.

Some physicians have noted that the rapid increase in the prevalence of overweight followed public health recommendations in the 1980s to eat low-fat diets. Low-fat diets usually translate into high-calorie, high-carbohydrate diets that, again, scrimp on protein, vitamins, and minerals.

Being overweight is the number-one risk factor for developing adult-onset (type 2) diabetes, and overweight children and teenagers now account for half of all new diagnoses of diabetes. The prevalence of type 2 diabetes among children has multiplied by an estimated fifteen to twenty-five times since 1980. Being overweight also increases the risk of hypertension, heart disease, gallstones, colon cancer, and (in men) stroke.

The Inflammation Syndrome Connection

The high-sugar and high-carbohydrate diets that lead to obesity raise glucose levels, and elevated glucose spontaneously generates large numbers of free radicals. These free radicals stimulate the inflammatory response, which can increase the risk of developing coronary artery disease, cancer, Alzheimer's, and many other diseases. In addition, abdominal fat cells secrete large quantities of pro-inflammatory interleukin-6 and C-reactive protein. In overweight and obese people, both of these substances help maintain a state of chronic inflammation.

Increases in body fat are often associated with disturbed hormone levels, such as elevated cortisol and insulin and decreased thyroid hormones. Sometimes figuring out which came first is like the chicken-or-the-egg story; however, being overweight leads to hormonal shifts that make it easy to gain still more weight. Because of the cell-regulating actions of weight-promoting hormones, it is very likely that they increase the activity of pro-inflammatory cytokines.

Standard Treatment

Conventional wisdom holds that people should eat fewer calories and exercise more to lose weight. Exercise helps because it creates more muscle cells, which burn calories for energy. But compelling research indicates that calories from protein and good fats are far better than those from carbohydrate-rich foods such as pasta, bread, and pizza. It makes no sense to build a diet around empty calories. Instead, follow a nutrient-dense diet such as the plan described in this book.

Nutrients That Can Help

The many fat-burning, fat-blocking, or carbohydrate-blocking supplements that are sold may help a small number of people, but they skirt the bottom-line issue: people cannot take a simple pill to compensate for bad eating habits. At best, it is naive to believe that supplements (or medications) can combat a diet full of high-calorie, high-carbohydrate refined foods.

Persuasive research by Harvard Medical School scientists has shown that diets rich in refined carbohydrates and carbohydrate-dense vegetables and grains increase CRP levels and inflammation. In the study, potatoes, breakfast cereals, white bread, muffins, and white rice were most strongly associated with elevated CRP levels. As with diabetes, it is essential that a person exercise the responsibility to choose healthier foods, such as those recommended in the AI Diet Plan. Such a diet should emphasize nutrient-dense lean meats (such as chicken and turkey), fish, and vegetables, while deemphasizing calorie-dense sugary foods and grain-based carbohydrates. The simple rule is to get as much diverse nutrition as possible in every bite of food. That is more easily accomplished with fish and vegetables than with pasta or pizza.

What Else Might Help?

A number of supplements might enhance weight reduction, but they are by themselves unlikely to burn off pounds of fat. Such supplements as alpha-lipoic acid, coenzyme Q_{10}, and carnitine play key roles in the cellular breakdown of glucose and fat. Supplements containing ephedra, a stimulant, may help as well—but they carry risks that include higher levels of anxiety and nervousness and increased blood pressure, and I do not recommend them.

Skin Disorders

What Are Skin Disorders?

Your skin is your body's largest and most direct interface with the world around you. As such, it is exposed to a wide variety of insults, including air pollution, chemicals, sunlight, bacteria, and viruses. Under these circumstances, a vast number of conditions can cause transitory or chronic inflammatory skin disorders. Only a few examples of inflammatory skin disorders will be described here as proof that anti-inflammatory nutrients can be beneficial. Among these disorders are contact dermatitis, sunburn, psoriasis, and eczema.

Causes

Dermatitis literally means "skin inflammation," and the term is usually interchangeable with *eczema*. Both are general descriptions, not specific diseases. Dermatitis can take a variety of forms anywhere on the body, such as itchiness, inflammation, swelling, and flaking skin. Many people consider dandruff a hair-related disorder, but it is actually a skin condition known as seborrheic dermatitis.

Contact dermatitis is often caused by direct handling of an irritating chemical. The body can often adapt to the exposure, which is what happens to people who regularly work with chemicals. After a number of years, however, many people pay a physiological price—complete intolerance of the chemical. Some types of contact dermatitis are also caused by specific naturally occurring compounds in a variety of foods. Dermatologists refer to this as "balsam-related contact dermatitis." The term comes from a plant extract called balsam of Peru, which contains allergenic substances that are also found in tomatoes, citrus, cola drinks, chocolate, and various spices (including vanilla).

Mild sunburn, known as erythema, is actually an inflammation of the skin. It is caused by damage from ultraviolet (UV) rays in sunlight, which split apart water molecules in cells and create free radicals. Tiny blood vessels rupture, and white blood cells respond to the damage. Regular sunburn or more severe sunburn can increase the long-term risk of getting skin cancers. That is because free radicals damage the DNA in skin cells.

Psoriasis is a chronic skin disease that often begins during a person's teenage years. It is characterized by thick, red skin patches. These patches are covered by white or silvery scales. These skin lesions itch, burn, crack, and sometimes bleed. About 15 percent of people with psoriasis also have arthritic joints, a condition known as psoriatic arthritis. Psoriasis tends to be worse during the winter months, when the air is drier and people have less exposure to sunlight.

Finally, wrinkling reflects age-related changes in the skin, including free-radical damage to the proteins forming skin and a thinning of the skin. Wrinkling can be accelerated by smoking and by excessive exposure to the sun.

How Common Are Skin Disorders?

Everyone experiences some type of dermatitis from time to time. Psoriasis, one of the most common chronic skin disorders, affects more than 7 million Americans. Many people enjoy the darker complexion afforded by a tan, but sun worshipers usually develop premature wrinkling and an increased risk of skin cancer, consequences of skin-cell damage from ultraviolet light.

The Inflammation Syndrome Connection

Research by Lester Packer, Ph.D., and Jens Thiele, M.D., of the University of California, Berkeley, has shown that the skin contains a reservoir of fatty acids and antioxidants. When the skin is exposed to ozone (a common air pollutant) or UV radiation, free radicals are generated, depleting these antioxidants and oxidizing fatty acids. UV-generated free-radical damage to the skin occurs in only two minutes. The inflammatory response happens much as it does elsewhere in the body, but it is far more visible. A blistering sunburn (or skin burns from chemicals and fire) is a sign of much more severe skin damage and cell death. Also important to note, skin levels of antioxidants decline with age, possibly increasing the rate of damage.

Standard Treatment

Treatments for psoriasis include corticosteroid drugs, both oral and topical. Corticosteroids are also used topically to treat many types of skin inflammation. Sunscreens can block some exposure to ultraviolet radiation, but they are often improperly used. For example, sunscreens protect the skin for short periods, and they are easily washed off.

Nutrients That Can Help

The classic signs of fatty-acid deficiency (omega-6, omega-3, or both) are dry and flaking skin. Such symptoms can develop when people are malnourished or eat low- or zero-fat diets. Eating fish and taking fish oil capsules can provide omega-3 fatty acids, and olive oil is an excellent source of omega-9 fatty acids. Adequate amounts of omega-6 fatty acids can be obtained in olive oil and raw nuts such as almonds or pumpkin seeds.

Several antioxidants have been shown to be helpful in reducing the effects of sunburn. Combined with omega-3 fatty acids, antioxidants can likely ease other forms of skin inflammation through an inside-out approach: take oral supplements and use a topical cream with antioxidants. Vitamin E is the body's principal fat-soluble antioxidant, meaning that it protects against free-radical damage in fatty parts of cells such as membranes. Topical applications are well absorbed through the skin, with some of the vitamin also entering the general circulation. In addition, topically applied vitamin E blocks UV damage to DNA. In a recent study Bernadette Eberlein-König, M.D., of the Technical University of Munich, measured how daily oral supplements of vitamin E (1,000 IU) and vitamin C (2,000 mg) increased resistance to UV rays. She found that subjects taking the vitamins were about 34 percent more resistant to sunburn, compared to people taking placebos.

Vitamin C also can also reduce the damaging effects of UV radiation. A study by Steven S. Traikovich, D.O., of Phoenix, Arizona, found that a vitamin C–containing lotion was able to lessen fine wrinkles, roughness, and skin tone, compared to a similar lotion without the vitamin. Vitamin C is essential for the body's production of collagen and elastin, two of the key proteins that form skin. In addition, several studies have found that beta-carotene supplements enhance the protective effects of sunscreen, illustrating the benefits of an inside-out approach to skin care.

Pycnogenol, a complex of antioxidant flavonoids extracted from the bark of French maritime pine trees, has been shown to reduce inflammation and, specifically, to protect skin cells. Laboratory experiments have shown that Pycnogenol decreases the activity of two genes, calgranulin A and B, which are overactive in psoriasis and some other skin disorders. Pycnogenol reduced the activity of calgranulin A and B by twenty-two times. Other researchers have shown that Pycnogenol helps prevent the breakdown of elastin from inflammation and free radicals.

What Else Might Help?

Like many herbs, chamomile *(Matricaria chamomilla)* is rich in antioxidants. In Germany, it has a rich history of use in treating skin disorders and is also found in many modern cosmetics. Allergist Holger Biltz, M.D., of Bad Honnef, Germany, found that a chamomile-containing cream alleviated reddening after UV exposure and reduced skin roughness. One high-quality line of chamomile-containing skin products is CamoCare, available at many natural foods stores and pharmacies. Green tea is also a powerful antioxidant and may be helpful in some skin disorders.

A wholesome diet, similar to the AI Diet Plan, can help preserve the skin. Australian researchers have reported that people who followed diets that consisted of large amounts of olive oil, fish, and vegetables experienced less facial wrinkling compared with people who ate more red meat, processed deli meats, soft drinks, and pastries.

Finally, it is paramount not to smoke tobacco products and not to be in the sun long enough to get sunburned. Smokers develop a particular type of facial wrinkling, which is related to their premature aging in general. Approximately fifteen minutes of sun exposure daily are sufficient for the body to make large amounts of vitamin D but not enough to result in sunburn (for most individuals). Longer sun exposure should be accompanied by the use of sunscreen or UV-blocking clothing.

A combination of omega-3 fish oils, gamma-linolenic acid, and vitamin D may be helpful in resolving eczema and psoriasis. Each of these nutrients can reduce inflammation, and they work better together. For difficult-to-treat toenail fungus, mix together either your topical prescription medication (e.g., ciclopirox) or tea tree oil with a small amount of DMSO (dimethylsulfone). You can dab this mixture on the affected toe. If you can get a clean syringe, use it to spray the solution under the affected nail, but be careful not to puncture the skin. DMSO helps transport other chemicals through the skin. Both tea tree oil and DMSO are available at most health food stores.

Sjögren's Syndrome

What Is Sjögren's Syndrome?

Sjögren's (pronounced *show-grins*) syndrome is usually associated with other autoimmune disorders, such as lupus and rheumatoid arthritis. Sjögren's initially targets fluid-secreting glands, and early symptoms often include dry eyes, mouth, and skin. The lack of saliva increases the likelihood of developing dental cavities, hoarseness, and oral yeast infections, and dry eyes can lead to visual problems. Sjögren's often results in an inflammation of the connective tissues that is symptomatically similar to that found in lupus and rheumatoid arthritis.

Causes

As with many complex disorders, conventional medicine has no official cause for Sjögren's syndrome; however, the leading risk factors include having some sort of rheumatic disease, being a woman, and being over age forty.

How Common Is Sjögren's Syndrome?

An estimated 1 million Americans have this disorder.

The Inflammation Syndrome Connection

There is a strong inflammatory undercurrent in Sjögren's syndrome. In addition to a progression to connective tissue, the kidneys, the liver, and the lungs can also become inflamed. As with fibromyalgia, many of the symptoms point to nutritional deficiencies or imbalances.

Standard Treatment

Conventional treatments of Sjögren's syndrome are geared toward easing symptoms. Medications include nonsteroidal anti-inflammatory drugs (NSAIDs), corticosteroids, and a variety of other drugs. Sometimes surgery is recommended for dry eyes.

Nutrients That Can Help

Dry eyes, skin, and mouth may suggest a deficiency of essential fatty acids, including EPA, DHA, and GLA. In fact, some research does point to an imbalance in these fatty acids in patients with Sjögren's syndrome. Supplementing with these fatty acids may help control symptoms. It is likely that other anti-inflammatory supplements and an anti-inflammatory diet will help reduce symptoms.

What Else Might Help?

Oral *Candida* yeast infections are common in people with Sjögren's syndrome. The presence of a localized yeast infection increases the risk of developing a systemic one, which can exacerbate symptoms. It is worthwhile discussing this possibility with your physician to determine whether a prescription antifungal drug (e.g., Lamisil) will reduce your symptoms.

AFTERWORD

Stay Healthy
for Life

Inflammation in response to an injury or an infection is a normal process that protects the body and promotes healing. It is also a transitory process that—again, normally—leaves behind no traces after the job is done. In contrast, chronic inflammation, whether it is mild or intense, is anything but normal. It is also a huge public health problem, based on the millions of people who suffer from its many manifestations and the hundreds of drugs marketed to treat it. Unfortunately, all of these drugs simply mask the most visible symptoms of inflammation. Drugs fail to address the underlying causes of chronic inflammation, and they often have dangerous side effects.

Part of the reason behind the widespread prevalence of inflammatory disorders is that many people never fully heal from their injuries, which can set the stage for long-term aches and pains and far more serious diseases. For example, the bangs and bruises of a college football player can slowly evolve into osteoarthritis. It is not only the initial damage to the joints that causes problems but also the consequences of sustained inflammation that the body did not throttle down. Similarly, people with serious head injuries, such as from falls, can throttle up inflammation in the brain that years later causes dementia.

Another reason for widespread inflammatory diseases in modern cultures is that the foods most people now eat do not support the healing

250

process and are in fact pro-inflammatory and antihealing. Since the 1970s, the pace of dietary changes has accelerated almost beyond comprehension, with nearly all of them having a negative effect on health. Most processed foods—those that come in boxes, cans, bottles, jars, and bags—have undergone intensive industrial manipulation. The result is almost always a food product that directly or indirectly promotes chronic inflammation. Incredibly, most of the ingredients in these processed foods would be unpalatable without the black magic of food technologists. For example, who on earth would ever use soybean oil as a salad dressing? It simply tastes awful. But when food companies add some sugar or salt, the tongue is tricked into sensing flavor in a pro-inflammatory food.

I always tell my nutrition-coaching clients that disease presents us with an opportunity. This is something I learned from a couple of cancer patients who told me that their disease was the "best thing" that ever happened to them. Of course, we can complain about the pain and limitations usually associated with disease, and many people do just that. But as with almost everything else in life, we have choices and those choices present us with opportunities.

In this respect, having an inflammatory disease is an opportunity to make our lives better. We can resolve the problem, minimize the chances of long-term disability, and transform the pain of inflammation into a powerful healing process. In this revised edition of *The Inflammation Syndrome*, I help you to do this. I have drawn on recent medical research to expand on my original recommendations for anti-inflammatory eating habits and supplements, while also trying to simplify those recommendations for practicality. Just as certain foods fuel the fires of inflammation, many others have the effect of dousing those flames. Armed with knowledge, it becomes easy to choose between healthy and unhealthy foods.

When *The Inflammation Syndrome* was first published in 2003, it was a bit ahead of its time. People had just started to connect the dots between inflammation and disease, particularly for diseases that had not traditionally been considered inflammatory (e.g., obesity, diabetes, and heart disease). It took a couple of years for the inflammation syndrome concept to gain "traction"—that is, for the scientific evidence to solidly catch up and for me to develop a following of readers. Since then, I have received e-mails from many people who said that the book transformed their lives and one from a man who stated that the book likely *saved* his life. Such feedback is more than just gratifying. It reminds me of the many people who are searching for real solutions for their health problems. I'm glad that I have been able to point them in the right direction. You, too, have the power to transform your health. I thank you for sharing your determination and your successes, and I encourage you to e-mail me your story at jchallem@aol.com.

Good health!

To save pages and trees, we have placed appendixes A and B and the medical references at www.inflammationsyndrome.com.

INDEX